Quality of Life in Asia

Volume 22

This series, the first of its kind, examines both the objective and subjective dimensions of life quality in Asia, especially East Asia. It unravels and compares the contours, dynamics and patterns of building nations by offering innovative works that discuss basic and applied research and emphasizing inter- and multi-disciplinary approaches to the various domains of life quality. The series appeals to a variety of fields in humanities, social sciences and other professional disciplines. Asia is the largest, most populous continent on Earth, and it is home to the world's most dynamic region, East Asia. In the past three decades, East Asia has been the most successful region in the world in expanding its economies and integrating them into the global economy, offering lessons on how poor countries, even with limited natural resources, can achieve rapid economic development. Yet while scholars and policymakers have focused on why East Asia has prospered, little has been written on how its economic expansion has affected the quality of life of its citizens. This series publish several volumes a year, either single or multiple-authored monographs or collections of essays.

Evelyn Tsz Yan Chan · Sunny H. Wong

Doctors' Work in the Public Hospital Sector in Hong Kong

The Construction of Meanings and Values in Medical Practice

Springer

Evelyn Tsz Yan Chan
CW Chu College
The Chinese University of Hong Kong
Shatin, NT, Hong Kong

Sunny H. Wong
Lee Kong Chian School of Medicine
Nanyang Technological University
Singapore, Singapore

ISSN 2211-0550 ISSN 2211-0569 (electronic)
Quality of Life in Asia
ISBN 978-981-96-6694-2 ISBN 978-981-96-6695-9 (eBook)
https://doi.org/10.1007/978-981-96-6695-9

This Springer imprint is published by the registered company Springer Nature Singapore Pte Ltd.
The registered company address is: 152 Beach Road, #21-01/04 Gateway East, Singapore 189721, Singapore

For Felicity and Nathan, who spurred me on

Acknowledgements Although we cannot thank them by name here, our deepest gratitude goes to the 27 public hospital doctors in this project who agreed to be interviewed, without whom this project would simply not have been possible.

The authors would also like to thank the following research assistants for their help with transcribing the interviews: Charlotte Chan, Vivien Chan, Pinky Lui, and Roxanne Shing.

The work for this project was fully supported by a grant from the Research Grants Council of Hong Kong (project number CUHK 14613721). The authors would like to extend their gratitude to the Council.

This book was inspired by a specialist consultation that the first author had with a public hospital doctor in Hong Kong, whose genuine care informed every aspect of that appointment. The consultation started her thoughts on what public hospital doctors might share about their work given the opportunity to discuss it, ultimately leading to the creation of this project. She would like to thank this doctor for providing the inspiration behind this book.

Competing Interests The authors have no competing interests to declare that are relevant to the content of this manuscript.

Contents

1 Introduction: Hong Kong Public Hospital Doctors' Work Narratives ... 1
1.1 Narrative Medicine ... 3
1.2 The Study, Its Aims, and Its Limitations ... 5
References ... 7

2 Narrative Interviews ... 11
2.1 Methodology ... 11
2.1.1 Background of the Interviewees ... 11
2.1.2 Interview Participation ... 12
2.1.3 Narrative Interview Method ... 13
2.2 Data Analysis ... 14
2.3 Results ... 18
2.3.1 Doctors' Reasons for Remaining in Public Hospital Work ... 18
2.3.2 Standards of Medical Work Set by Doctors ... 49
2.3.3 Work Problems in Public Hospitals ... 62
2.3.4 Personal Problems Caused by Work ... 75
2.3.5 Strategies to Cope with Work Demands ... 84
2.4 Final Remarks ... 94
References ... 94

3 Concluding Reflections ... 95
3.1 Work as a Public Good ... 97
3.2 Work as Part of Communities ... 99
3.3 Negotiating the Ideal of the "Good" Doctor ... 102
3.4 Towards an Ethics of Care: Empathy and Emotions ... 105
3.5 Closing Remarks ... 110
References ... 111

Chapter 1
Introduction: Hong Kong Public Hospital Doctors' Work Narratives

Abstract This Introduction lays out the study's background, research aims, and rationale. Using collected interview narratives, this study explores how public hospital sector doctors in Hong Kong understand their work and careers, and the meanings and values they construct and ascribe to these. The Introduction situates the study in the context of Hong Kong and in existing literature on the use of narrative in the medical field. The use of interview narratives, instead of other types of data, is crucial to this study's examination of doctors' experiences and struggles in their particular work context. The Introduction argues that this has educational value for a wide variety of audiences.

Keywords The public hospital sector in Hong Kong · Narrative medicine · Hong Kong public hospital doctors' work narratives · Interviews with Hong Kong public hospital doctors · Interpreting medical practice through narrative · Human values in the medical profession · Meanings and values in the medical profession · Narrative research in the health sciences

Public hospitals in Hong Kong face a number of well-documented challenges that have a big impact on the working conditions of medical personnel in these institutions. These challenges include a rapidly ageing population, rising costs, long waiting times for patients, insufficient service slots and hospital beds especially at periodic peak usage times, and a shortage of medical personnel as these move to the private sector in search of less pressing work conditions or higher pay (Lam, 2017; Lieu, 2006). Although at first glance these problems would seem similar to those afflicting other developed places, the degree to which these problems exist in Hong Kong makes the Hong Kong public hospital a particularly charged and challenging environment to work in.

To understand this, and to understand the value of this book's examination of public hospital doctors' narratives of work within this context, we need to provide a brief overview of the public healthcare sector in Hong Kong. In Hong Kong, healthcare services are provided by both a public system that is almost entirely subsidized by the government (Health bureau, 2023; Lam, 2024; Wong et al., 2015),

E. T. Y. Chan and S. Wong, *Doctors' Work in the Public Hospital Sector in Hong Kong*, Quality of Life in Asia 22, https://doi.org/10.1007/978-981-96-6695-9_1

and a private system where almost the entire cost is borne by users themselves. Services in the public healthcare sector are offered at nominal fees to the patient even as it delivers overall outcomes that are amongst the best in the world, including the longest average lifespan and one of the lowest infant mortality rates in the world (Ramesh, 2012). This makes public healthcare services available to everyone in a society that is one of the most unequal in the world in terms of income distribution: Hong Kong's Gini index in 2016 was 53.9, putting it in fifth place in terms of inequality in family income (*The World Factbook*, n.d.).

The Hospital Authority is the main provider of public healthcare services in Hong Kong, and governs 43 public hospitals, 49 specialist out-patient clinics, and 74 general out-patient clinics, located in seven location clusters (Hospital Authority, 2025). Public hospitals deliver approximately 90% of inpatient hospital care in Hong Kong, with the private sector responsible for the rest (Wong et al., 2015; Wu et al., 2023). Conversely, the public sector provides around 30% of outpatient services, with the private sector in charge of 70% of such services (Wu et al., 2023). Although the private sector caters for the bulk of outpatient services in Hong Kong, the heavy inpatient load for public hospitals in Hong Kong has created an extremely overstretched public hospital sector, with prolonged wait times for patients (Zou & Chen, 2022). This is aggravated by the serious shortage of doctors in the public sector (Health Bureau, 2021), with the public and private healthcare sectors each employing around half of the total number of doctors in Hong Kong (Information Services Department, 2024) despite the bulk of inpatient care falling on public hospitals. The high rate of doctors moving from public hospitals to the private sector, attracted by higher pay and better working conditions, contributes further to a chronic workforce shortage in the public hospital sector, which in turn further worsens working conditions and waiting times there (Tsui & Fong, 2018). In 2021–2022, for instance, doctors having 11 to 16 years of experience—which is when doctors have obtained their specialist qualifications—comprised the largest group leaving the public sector, followed by those with one to six years of experience (Mycroft, 2023). Despite government measures designed to alleviate the systemic challenges faced by public hospitals in Hong Kong, such as the implementation of the Voluntary Health Insurance Scheme in order to take some pressure off the public health sector, these challenges are set to worsen in the near future as the population continues to age and the extent of the shortage of doctors is projected to worsen (Research Office, 2024).

This book is the first to examine doctors' subjective experiences of work in this environment. Work is made meaningful not just by its material rewards, but also by the values ascribed to it by practitioners. These values drive practitioners forward despite adverse conditions and shape their work and careers. Work for doctors in public hospitals in Hong Kong combines structured professional codes of conduct, extensive contact with the public on whom their work has a large impact, and a stressful, high-stakes environment where they are pressed for time and resources. This combination makes the question of what human values and meanings sustain, nourish, and improve their work an especially valuable area of research, creating important insights into their work.

This book explores narratives told by some of these doctors of their work in this context as they encounter and process "those moments of greatest human drama (birth, illness, injury, suffering, disease, death)" (McLellan, 1997) in it. Using narrative interviews with 27 medical doctors in Hong Kong who have worked in the public hospital sector for approximately 10 years or more, the study investigates how public hospital sector doctors in Hong Kong understand their work and careers, analyses the meanings and values they construct and ascribe to these, and examines how they have coped with hardships and crises. Revealing and studying the meanings and values that underpin such doctors' work as expressed through their own narratives means that this study can serve several purposes. It can provide guidance for medical students as they stand poised to start their own work journey. It can inform the practice of other doctors as they navigate similar issues in their own work. It can provide an alternative reference for medical administrators as they seek to tackle the problems the sector faces, even if, as explained later in this chapter, this book is not a study on public health policy. And it can offer the public a rare window into public hospital doctors' work, shedding light on its human dimensions, and increasing their understanding of a profession that can otherwise seem closed off to outsiders, but which is so crucial to people's lives and wellbeing.

1.1 Narrative Medicine

This book's choice in using narrative, or the arrangement of "human experiences into temporally meaningful episodes" (Polkinghorne, 1988, p. 1), emphasizes participants' subjective and lived experience of their work. Narrative has been recognized as essential in helping people make sense of lived experience and constructing their sense of self by going beyond what Jerome Bruner (1986) and Donald Polkinghorne (1988) have referred to as paradigmatic, or logico-scientific, knowledge. In medicine, the narrative dimension helps to foreground the human, interpretive paradigm of medicine, which theories of clinical management, in their focus on the scientific paradigm of medical diagnosis and treatment, tend to undervalue. Chapter 2 in this book goes into more detail about what elements of narrative this study draws on, but this section for now discusses the relevance to this study of how the narratives we tell about ourselves allow us to "recognize what parts we play in one another's lives and how entailed we are in our shared creation of meaning" (Charon, 2006, p. 10). Through such narratives, "We get to know ourselves as a result of the vision of others," and become "able to donate ourselves as instruments of others' learning" (Charon, 2006, p. 10).

The focus on narrative within medicine has led to the disciplinary field of what Rita Charon (2006) has called narrative medicine. One approach within this broad field is to assign and explore narrative elements in clinical judgement and situations by the researcher who sees how these are "narratively based," or as Marcia Day Childress (2017) has put it, "'storying' language in and about medicine" using approaches "borrow[ed] from literary study—close reading [...], analysis, and interpretation" (pp. 273–74). Another is to ask and teach doctors and doctors-to-be to render their thoughts and experiences into narratives, which has become an established practice in medical training at some universities. For instance, Childress writes of her own experience teaching medical students to write narratives that "physicians know, remember, and learn from patients and practice situations *as stories*. They process clinical experience as Charon's narrative knowledge—as 'pearls' or lessons, epiphanies, or cautionary tales" (p. 275). The explicit "storying"—or rendering into narratives—of their experience, when conducted by doctors and doctors-to-be, allows them to be more reflective about their practice, to, for instance, "elucidat[e] moral lessons" (Childress, 2017, p. 276) through the writing process.

In line with this second approach, the field of narrative medicine has expanded into researchers' use of narratives by doctors, collected through interviews as primary research data, to provide further insight into doctors' work experiences. Some studies, for instance, have explored doctors' written narratives to address exploratory questions on a variety of topics, such as on everyday ethics (Avrahami, 2011). Other studies have used interview narratives to answer focused research questions. To name just a few examples here, this includes studies on what interview narratives reveal about emotion regulation by doctors (Lundin et al., 2018), ideals of competence (Crowe & Brugha, 2018), hierarchy and emotions in doctors' relations (Crowe et al., 2017), and hospital doctors' views on their wellbeing during the recent COVID pandemic (Creese et al., 2021). One of the very few Hong Kong-based studies also using interview narratives is an investigation into migrant doctors' construction of professional identity as evidenced in semi-structured interviews (Lazzaro-Salazar & Zayts, 2023).

However, although individual doctors' memoirs or non-fictional books based on doctors' own clinical experience exist—for instance Oliver Sacks's *The Mind's Eye*, Kate Scannell's *Death of the Good Doctor: Lessons from the Heart of the AIDS Epidemic*, and Abraham Verghese's *My Own Country: A Doctor's Story*—book-length studies using interview narratives as the basis, as is the case in the present study, are somewhat rarer in medical humanities or narrative medicine research. Most of the book-length research works on the narratives that doctors' work generates have led not to published outputs of narratives, but to methodological and theoretical discussions of the narrative underpinnings of medical practice. For instance, Kathryn Montgomery's *Doctors' Stories: The Narrative Structure of Medical Knowledge* and *How Doctors Think: Clinical Judgment and the Practice of Medicine* are major texts in the field that are not collections of narratives by doctors, but meta-narrative discussions: they discuss and argue for the many narrative aspects of doctors' work.

The present study is a combination of some of the approaches outlined above. First, it is premised on the same assumption as that taken in the cited works above: that narrative is an important way to process, reflect on, and reveal the lived experience of medical work. This applies to the interviewed doctors in this study as the meanings and values of their work are established and consolidated through the interview narratives that they chose to tell and defined their work and work identities by. Although the doctors this study interviewed were not professional writers, the study put them in the position—at least for the duration of the interview—of being writers of the personal values and significances of their practice. Second, like the articles cited, this study examines interview narratives for the specific research aim of exploring doctors' subjective understanding of their work in public hospitals in Hong Kong. Third, instead of presenting the results of the research aims in a truncated way—as would be necessary for an article-length study—this study devotes the bulk of the space of this book in Chap. 2 to allowing doctors' voices to be heard largely in their own (translated) words. In this way, this study partially looks to the doctors' memoirs cited in the last paragraphs, working on the basis that the stories doctors tell of their work experience have a narrative appeal to a wider audience. Reducing narratives to a very brief summary of results may strip them of much of their power, while avoiding excessive reduction can help preserve their "compelling form" (Hurwitz, 2000, p. 2088). The extensive quotations form the narratives in this study allow them to better resonate with a variety of audiences—whether these are medical students, doctors, educators, administrators, or the general public—on a deeper level than a mere summary of results would provide. In addition, the greater space a full book allowed us, in contrast with the shorter length of an article, meant that a much longer and more comprehensive list of themes could be used to express the results. The next section will provide more details of this study's approach as a prelude to the methodological discussion in Chap. 2, as well as of limitations to the study.

1.2 The Study, Its Aims, and Its Limitations

The present study, as mentioned, is based on interviews on their work with 27 medical doctors who have worked in the public hospital sector in Hong Kong for approximately 10 years or more. It examines how these doctors understand their work experience, focusing on what values and meanings underpin their medical practice. As Chap. 2 explains in more detail, the interview narratives were thematically analysed, aiming to demonstrate and explore:

- How public hospital doctors in Hong Kong understood their work and their careers;
- What meanings and values sustained their work;
- What aspects of their work had proved beneficial to them, and had enabled them to find sustaining meaning;
- And how they had coped with hardships and crises in their work.

The account of complete narrative structure by Labov and Waletzky (1967) contains the six structural elements of the abstract (a summary of the topic), orientation (in terms of time, place, and context), complicating action, evaluation, resolution, and coda (relating the events back to present). Some of these elements match the aims of the study outlined above, where the orientation aligns with the examined context of doctors' work in public hospitals in Hong Kong, evaluation ties to doctors' subjective meaning-creation in their work, and complicating action and resolution correspond to their work challenges and coping methods. Labov and Waletzky's model provides a frame of reference for narrative structure, but this study's data will not be strictly mapped onto this model, as it is not necessary for the study's aims, as will be further discussed in Chap. 2. Instead, the broad approach of seeing narrative as, in a general sense, a subjective, interpretive way "of ordering experience" and "constructing reality" that is embedded in "the particulars of experience located in time and place" and in particular contexts guides the study's aims and analysis (Moniz et al., 2021, p. 27).

Having said that, there are several caveats to be made with regard to the scope of the study. This study uses interview narratives as a data source. It does so without studying narrative itself as a practice, or focusing on the theoretical or philosophical bases for the phenomenon or use of narrative in medicine. Although this study is based on narrative production by doctors, it did not ask or instruct doctors to be aware of the narrative underpinnings of their work practice and to use such knowledge to inform the narratives they produced. The educational potential for the narrating doctor in the course of constructing the narratives was therefore not one of the foci, as it is in some of the scholarship cited in the previous section. However, this does not preclude the educational potential of the narratives on other people, and as mentioned, it is part of this study's goal to inform others of the experiences of medical work, including other medical staff, whose future medical practice may in turn be informed in the process.

In addition, the present study neither focuses on public healthcare policy, nor is primarily directed at informing it. The study's emphasis is on how Hong Kong public hospital doctors understand their work and work identities, and on the subjective dimensions of doctors' experience, and not on recommendations on a way forward for the Hong Kong health sector. The study therefore does not seek to provide solutions to the issues of the Hong Kong public hospital sector that serve as a background to the narratives of work. Nevertheless, the context of the Hong Kong public hospital is important because this study wishes to uncover doctors' subjective experiences as based in this particular environment, where such experience has been shaped and is located. Therefore, the study can be read as complementary and able to be contextualized within, yet distinct from, previous works on the Hong Kong health system from public health and policy perspectives.[1]

The contribution this book makes thus lies in several aspects. The first, as mentioned, is that it is a book-length study that quotes extensively from interviews with the doctors. This puts it in contrast with books that aim to provide more theoretical discussions on the use of narrative in medicine, or autobiographical narratives written from the perspective of a single narrating doctor. This also puts it in contrast with the article-length studies cited in the last section, which are methodologically

---

[1] Some prominent examples of such works, both recent and from earlier periods, include books on the Hong Kong health system, such as Robin Gauld and Derek Gould's *The Hong Kong Health Sector* and Gabriel M. Leung and John Bacon-Shone's edited volume *Hong Kong's Health System: Book Subtitle: Reflections, Perspectives and Visions*, and books that engage with particular topics relevant to Hong Kong healthcare, such as Vincent Tin Sing Law and Ben Yuk Fai Fong's edited volume *Ageing with Dignity in Hong Kong and Asia.*

more closely aligned with this study in that this study also uses doctors' interview narratives to answer specific research questions on doctors' work experiences and identities, but which do not have much space to represent these narratives in interviewees' own words. Most importantly, there are very few studies that use narratives as research material on Hong Kong healthcare, and to the authors' knowledge, no book-length studies on doctors' narratives of work exist within this context.

The extended quotations allow a deeper understanding of the lived experience of Hong Kong public hospital doctors than hitherto provided. Such deeper understanding can facilitate debate and reflection on such work from an alternative angle, and by a wider variety of stakeholders. Existing doctors can benefit from exploring their colleagues' ways of thinking about their work. Medical students can reflect on some of the struggles and rewards that may lie ahead of them in a public hospital career. And the public can gain insight into doctors' perspectives about their work that rarely, if ever, make it into a medical consultation. These outcomes will not readily lead to specific solutions to problems plaguing the sector, yet they can re-engage debates on such problems from the specific and relatively less explored perspective of the public hospital doctor's reflections and thoughts.

The next chapter further explains the methodology of the study. It also presents and discusses the results of the thematic analysis of the interview narratives, providing an overview of the values and meanings doctors ascribed to their work without sacrificing the opportunity to hear their first-person accounts because of the extensive interview quotations used. These interview passages capture the many moments, experiences, and reflections that comprise doctors' work. The chapter is the longest in the book, where we were able to make full use of the fact that this is a book-length and not an article-length study to lay out a much more extensive and detailed list of themes, with smaller distinctions between themes than we would have made had we had less space available to us. The final chapter of this book will examine and discuss the major thematic strands that can be distilled from these themes and issues, and what these can further reveal about the challenges that doctors face, and the areas in their work that would benefit from recognizing improving, or supporting.

References

Avrahami, E. (2011). Positive wrongngs: Reading doctors' narratives on ordinary ethics. *Literature and Medicine 29*(2), 325–354. https://doi.org/10.1353/lm.2011.0327

Bruner, J. (1986). *Actual minds, possible worlds*. Harvard University Press.

Charon, R. (2006). *Narrative medicine: Honoring the stories of illness*. Oxford University Press.

Childress, M. D. (2017). From doctors' stories to doctors' stories, and back again. *AMA Journal of Ethics*, *19*(3), 272–280. https://journalofethics.ama-assn.org/article/doctors-stories-doctors-stories-and-back-again/2017-03

Creese, J., Byrne, J.-P., Conway, E., Barrett, E., Prihodova, L., & Humphries, N. (2021). "We all really need to just take a breath": Composite narratives of hospital doctors' well-being during the COVID-19 pandemic. *International Journal of Environmental Research and Public Health*, *18*(4), 2051. https://doi.org/10.3390/ijerph18042051

Crowe, S., & Brugha, R. (2018). "We've all had patients who've died …": Narratives of emotion and ideals of competence among junior doctors. *Social Science & Medicine, 215*, 152–159. https://doi.org/10.1016/j.socscimed.2018.08.037

Crowe, S., Clarke, N., & Brugha, R. (2017). "You do not cross them": Hierarchy and emotion in doctors' narratives of power relations in specialist training. *Social Science & Medicine, 186*, 70–77. https://doi.org/10.1016/j.socscimed.2017.05.048

Gauld, R., & Gould, D. (2002). *The Hong Kong health sector*. The Chinese University Press.

Health Bureau. (2021). *Medical registration (amendment) bill 2021*. https://www.healthbureau.gov.hk/download/press_and_publications/otherinfo/210500_amendments_mro/e_legco_brief.pdf

Health Bureau. (2023, January 30). The healthcare challenges in Hong Kong. *Primary healthcare blueprint*. https://www.primaryhealthcare.gov.hk/bp/en/blueprint-2/

Hospital Authority. (2025). *Clusters, hospitals & institutions*. https://www.ha.org.hk/visitor/ha_visitor_index.asp?Content_ID=10036&Lang=ENG

Hurwitz B. (2000). Narrative and the practice of medicine. *Lancet, 356*(9247), 2086–2089. https://www.thelancet.com/journals/lancet/article/PIIS0140-6736(00)03412-7

Information Services Department. (2024, June 26). *Govt eases public hospitals' burden*. News.gov.hk. https://www.news.gov.hk/eng/2024/06/20240626/20240626_164712_292.html

Labov, W., & Waletzky, W. (1967). Narrative analysis: Oral versions of personal experience. In J. Helms (Ed.), *Essays on the verbal and visual Arts* (pp. 12–44). University of Washington Press.

Lam, A. H. Y. (2017). Strategies of Hong Kong's healthcare system in aging population. In *Official conference proceedings of the Asian conference on aging & gerontology*. The University of Hong Kong. https://papers.iafor.org/wp-content/uploads/papers/agen2017/AGEN2017_36030.pdf

Lam, D. T. Y. (2024). Three critical elements of sustainable healthcare. In *Building a sustainable healthcare system for Hong Kong* (pp. 11–26). The Hong Kong institute of Asia-Pacific Studies, The Chinese University of Hong Kong. https://www.hkiaps.cuhk.edu.hk/wp-content/uploads/2024/07/PRR07.pdf

Law, V. T. S., & Fong, B. Y. F. (Eds.) (2022). *Ageing with dignity in Hong Kong and Asia*. Springer.

Lazzaro-Salazar, M., & Zayts, O. (2023). Migrant doctors' narratives about patients: A study of professional identity in Chile and Hong Kong. *Narrative Inquiry, 33*(1), 153–175. https://doi.org/10.1075/ni.21038.laz

Leung, G. M., & Bacon-Shone, J. (Eds.) (2006). *Hong Kong's health system: Reflections, perspectives and visions*. The Hong Kong University Press.

Lieu, G. (2006). Quality indicators and health targets. In G. M. Leung & J. Bacon-Shone (Eds.), *Hong Kong's health System: Reflections, perspectives and visions* (pp. 303–326). Hong Kong University Press. https://www.jstor.org/stable/j.ctt1xwg30.22

Lundin, R. M., Bashir, K., Bullock, A., Kostov, C. E., Mattick, K. L., Rees, C. E., & Monrouxe, L. V. (2018). "I'd been like freaking out the whole night": Exploring emotion regulation based on junior doctors' narratives. *Advances in Health Sciences Education, 23*, 7–28. https://doi.org/10.1007/s10459-017-9769-y

McLellan, M. F. (1997). Literature and medicine: Physician-writers. *The Lancet, 349*(9051), 564–567. https://doi.org/10.1016/S0140-6736(97)80120-1

Moniz, T., Costella, J., Golafshani, M., Watling, C., & Lingard, L. (2021). Bringing narratives from physicians, patients and caregivers together: A scoping review of published research. *Medical Humanities, 47*(1), 27–37. https://mh.bmj.com/content/47/1/27

Montgomery, K. (1991). *Doctors' stories: The narrative structure of medical knowledge*. Princeton University Press.

Montgomery, K. (2006). *How doctors think: Clinical judgment and the practice of medicine*. Oxford University Press.

Mycroft, C. (2023, August 20). Hong Kong health minister raises concerns over public hospital doctors going private after specialising. *South China Morning Post*. https://www.scmp.com/news/hong-kong/health-environment/article/3231693/hong-kong-health-minister-raises-concerns-over-public-hospital-doctors-going-private-after

Polkinghorne, D. (1988). *Narrative knowing and the human sciences*. State University of New York Press.

Ramesh, M. (2012). Health care reform in Hong Kong: The politics of liberal non-democracy. *The Pacific Review, 25*(4), 455–471. https://doi.org/10.1080/09512748.2012.685095

Research Office. (2024). *Shortage of doctors in Hong Kong* (ISSH32/2024). Legislative Council Secretariat. https://app7.legco.gov.hk/rpdb/en/file.aspx?id=7437bd1b2d614f5faf8cf00b349b3c11&type=pdf&lang1=en&lang2=en

The World Factbook. *Gini Index coefficient—Distribution of family income*. https://www.cia.gov/the-world-factbook/field/gini-index-coefficient-distribution-of-family-income/country-comparison/

Tsui, Y. M., & Fong, B. Y. (2018). Waiting time in public hospitals: Case study of total joint replacement in Hong Kong. *Public Administration and Policy, 21*(2), 120–133. https://www.emerald.com/insight/content/doi/10.1108/pap-10-2018-009/full/html

Wong, E. L., Yeoh, E. K., Chau, P. Y., Yam, C. H., Cheung, A. W., & Fung, H. (2015). How shall we examine and learn about public-private partnerships (PPPs) in the health sector? Realist evaluation of PPPs in Hong Kong. *Social Science & Medicine, 147*, 261–269. https://doi.org/10.1016/j.socscimed.2015.11.012

Wu, Y., Wang, D. Y., Zhao, S., Wang, M. H., Wong, E. L., & Yeoh, E. K. (2023). Emergency department use across income groups following an increase in cost-Sharing. *JAMA Network Open, 6*(8), Article e2329577. https://doi.org/10.1001/jamanetworkopen.2023.29577

Zou, Y., & Chen, J. (2022). The feedback loop between the demand for voluntary private insurance and the burden of healthcare system: an explanatory system dynamics model of Hong Kong. *International Journal of Health Policy and Management, 11*(12), 3040–3051. https://www.ijhpm.com/article_4277.html

Chapter 2
Narrative Interviews

Abstract Narratives of work by medical doctors in the public hospital sector in Hong Kong, who had accumulated approximately 10 years or more of work experience there, were collected for this study through the use of partially structured interviews. This chapter explains the methodology of the data collection process. It then presents and discusses the results of the thematic analysis of the interview narratives, showing the various ideals and meanings doctors ascribed to their work, the benefits they saw in their work, the standards of work they set themselves, the challenges they faced, and the coping strategies they used. The chapter uses extensive interview quotations to allow doctors' own voices to come through. These direct quotations reveal the spectrum of reflections, experiences, and moments—whether small and fleeting, or lasting and profound—that shaped their journey.

Keywords The public hospital sector in Hong Kong · Narrative medicine · Hong Kong public hospital doctors' work narratives · Interviews with Hong Kong public hospital doctors · Interpreting medical practice through narrative · Human values in the medical profession · Meanings and values in the medical profession · The lived experience of medical practice · Reflexivity in medical practice · Narrative research in the health sciences · Quality of life and work for medical doctors

2.1 Methodology

2.1.1 Background of the Interviewees

From March to October 2022, 27 doctors who had been working in Hong Kong public hospitals for approximately 10 years or more participated in this study's interviews (Fig. 2.1). The length of their careers meant that interviewees had all passed their specialist training and examinations, accumulated extensive experience in this setting, and could discuss their work in depth. To ensure that responses were not clustered around doctors from only a few select specialties, participants from 16 different medical specialties as recognized by the Medical Council in Hong Kong

E. T. Y. Chan and S. Wong, *Doctors' Work in the Public Hospital Sector in Hong Kong*, Quality of Life in Asia 22, https://doi.org/10.1007/978-981-96-6695-9_2

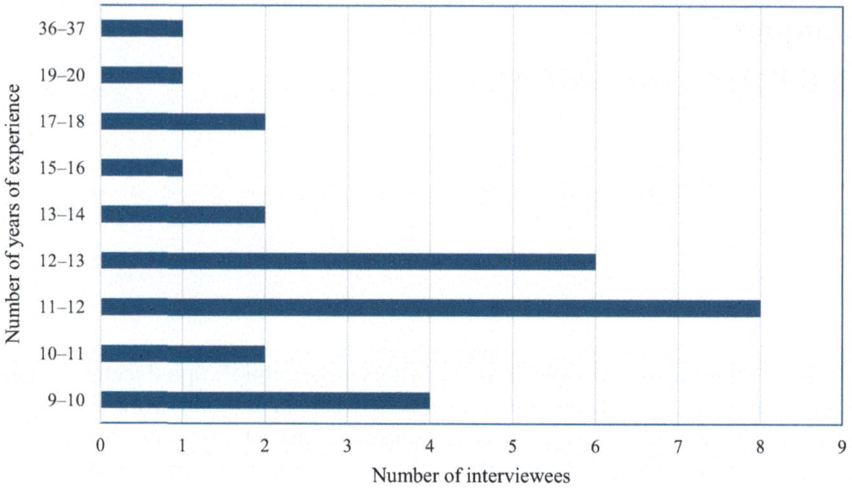

Fig. 2.1 Interviewees' number of years of public hospital work experience in Hong Kong

were interviewed. 12 of the participants were female, and 15 were male. All the participants were ethnic Chinese. Most had received their qualifying medical degree in Hong Kong.

Doctors in Hong Kong tend to move around various public hospitals throughout their career as dictated by staffing and training needs, and may also be affiliated with more than one public hospital. As such, current hospital affiliation was not considered to have a bearing on the study design, and was not taken into account during the participant recruitment process.

2.1.2 Interview Participation

The first few interviewees were invited to participate in the study by the second author, who had himself been a public hospital doctor in Hong Kong. Subsequent to this initial stage, the main participant recruitment method used was snowball sampling, which was the most workable and practicable for this study's purposes. We asked participants to recommend any further interviewees, in particular those who were of a different specialty, who might be willing to share their thoughts and experiences in an interview. Participants then obtained consent from the doctors they recommended before we initiated contact. This referral process ensured a high response rate in a group of participants who would have otherwise been difficult to recruit for in-depth interviews because of their very busy schedules.

Using snowball sampling means the recruitment process was not random, and the study's results cannot claim to represent all public hospital doctors' views. However, representativeness is not an aim of this study, which is not a survey. The study does not seek to provide a comprehensive and overarching picture of all relevant aspects of doctors' public hospital work in Hong Kong. Rather, as explained in the Introduction, the study aims to explore how individual public hospital doctors in Hong Kong understood their work and their careers, and what meanings and values sustained their work. Therefore, identifying interviewees with deep personal insights and values was more important for data quality than ensuring random participant recruitment.

Despite its main limitation of not providing a representative sample, snowball sampling aligned well with the study's theoretical approach. Grounded in the interpretivist paradigm of qualitative, and specifically narrative, research, the focus was on participants' subjective experiences and how they constructed them through narrative. This subjective, narrative approach offers detailed individual views rarely presented in Hong Kong studies, providing valuable insights into doctors' lived experiences. This theoretical approach also informed the interview format and the method of thematic analysis implemented, as will be discussed in the next sections.

2.1.3 Narrative Interview Method

We conducted partially structured interviews, with the goal to elicit doctors' individual narratives of work with sufficient structure so that different interviews could be compared, but at the same time to allow ample flexibility for in-depth exploration of any issues that arose throughout the interview. Set questions were combined with follow-up questions on topics that were discussed. These follow-up questions were raised when interviewees stopped talking after each set question. The overall model applied was then the "lightly structured depth interview" particularly suited to the biographic narrative (Wengraf, 2001): "lightly structured" with partially set questions, and containing "depth" where the complexities of the research topic—in this case doctors' meaning- and value-construction—were delved into during the interview.

The set questions outlined below encouraged the creation of subjective meaning rather than extracting objective, factual information. In devising the set questions, it was our conscious choice not to ask participants to share their views on narrow issues, or on a list of topics on public sector medical work. Instead, we asked questions linked to some of the core attributes of narratives: those of context, conflict, and reconciliation or resolution (or coping), as based on the influential account of narrative structure by Labov and Waletzky (1967) mentioned in the previous chapter. These questions allowed doctors to frame their subjective responses to their work and its context, resulting in unique narratives by each participant. The first three questions were exploratory and encouraged individual narrative production of participants' subjective experience of work. The fourth question captured any conscious values and work experiences beyond the ones already mentioned that interviewees considered to underpin their medical practices. The last question asked doctors to narrate experiences that had a particularly lasting impact on their work.

The set interview questions were:

- How have your feelings and attitudes towards your profession changed since you first started working in the public hospital sector in Hong Kong?
- Could you talk about what being a doctor in a public hospital means to you? Has this also changed over time?
- How do you cope with the demands placed on you in the public hospital sector?
- Could you talk about the values that sustain you in your work? How were these formed?
- Could you talk about specific experiences in your work that have influenced the values or meanings that you ascribe to your work?

The interviews lasted from around 30 min—the anticipated duration communicated to participants—to almost two hours, depending on interviewees' availability and the conversational flow.

2.2 Data Analysis

The interviews were transcribed verbatim and subsequently analyzed thematically. Similar to the use of the partially structured interview, thematic analysis, which identifies common themes across narratives, provides a good balance between yielding specific insights into the individual narrative and exploring shared ideas. In particular, it is a highly effective way of organizing, analyzing, and representing large amounts of narrative data, with the resulting shared semantic units identified able to more clearly and systematically address the research aims.

However, since thematic analysis focuses predominantly on the content of narratives, this may come at the cost of understating other ways of looking at narrative, such as narrative as chronological progression, or as a performative collaboration between the interviewee, the interviewer, and any relevant social contexts. Although these alternative ways of looking at narrative did not provide the foundation for the data analysis method used in this study, they nevertheless appeared at times as part of the results of thematic analysis. For instance, some themes included chronological progression (such as "further training and enhanced learning" and "increasing autonomy and ownership with seniority"), while other themes were grounded in a performative way of looking at doctors' roles (such as "compassionate, effective communication in care"). Rather than seeing thematic analysis as precluding other approaches to narrative analysis, therefore, we saw it as including some of these other aspects without putting the main emphasis on them. This is especially the case since there are no rigid boundaries around content vis-à-vis other narrative aspects: content does not exclude these other aspects, but rather also contains them.

In this study, we created themes through the iterative reading and processing of the interview data. Themes were semantic units within the interview data that were sufficiently discrete to be defined clearly. As mentioned in the Introduction, because of the space accorded by this book-length, instead of article-length, study, we could examine a much more extensive and detailed list of themes, and make smaller distinctions between themes than we otherwise would have. We drew up lists of themes and redrafted them while the interview data was interpreted and re-interpreted. We also adjusted themes to ensure distinctness and definition, even as there were connections and inevitably some degree of overlap between them. Partial overlap could also occur due to interview quotations that needed to be read in their entirety for narrative clarity and understanding, but which might contain some smaller narrative elements that could fall under another theme. In such a case, we either decided which theme was the most suitable for the interview quotation as a whole, and assigned it to that theme in the final version, or we separated the smaller narrative elements from the longer quotation and assigned them into their respective themes.

Thematic analysis occurred in four stages. In the first stage, we read through the interview transcripts several times in their entirety. In the second stage, we conducted thematic coding using NVIVO while reading all the interview transcripts once again. The emerging list of groups, categories, and themes, all called "codes" for short in this section, was continuously added to and modified throughout the coding process, until the first draft of the list of codes was arrived at. In the third stage, all the coded interview quotations were reread and their fit with their assigned codes reconfirmed, while the quotations that had been mapped onto multiple themes were assigned their final theme to which they showed the strongest relevance. Codes were adjusted throughout this stage to clarify the boundaries between them, while taking into account that a limited degree of overlap even between final codes is inevitable in thematic analysis. In the fourth stage, all codes and their interview quotations were compiled into one single document by editing the interview quotations and translating Cantonese interview quotations into English, with the editing method used described in the next paragraph. Further adjustment of code titles occurred at this stage.

In a study that emphasizes participants' subjective views and voices, it was important that these were not obscured by excessive editing. Minor editing of the interview quotations took the form of the elision of repeated single words or brief phrases (such as the repetition of "perhaps" across several consecutive clauses or sentences), small lexical and non-lexical hesitations, single filler words or short filler phrases (for instance "that is," very commonly used to link sentences together in spoken Cantonese), and single words and brief phrases that turned into rephrasing and restarts. Minor grammatical mistakes, common across all speech production, were also corrected (for instance subject-object agreement in English interviews). In order not to impede the flow of the representation of the interview quotations, such minor editing is not indicated in the final quotations shown in this chapter. However, the presence of elided speech segments that fell outside the scope of such minor editing are indicated using ellipses in square brackets ("[…]"), to be distinguished from inherent speech breaks and hesitations by the speakers themselves, which are indicated using ellipses without square brackets ("…").

We struck a balance between literal and idiomatic translation when translating Cantonese speech into English text, so that the end result could capture as much as the original speech as possible while also approximating natural speech. Translated Cantonese interview quotations are indicated using "[CAN]" at the end of each quotation, whereas English interview quotations are not marked. If interviewees used English words or phrases in an otherwise Cantonese interview, these were put in quotation marks within the interview quotation. These instances can generally be distinguished from when doctors themselves used direct speech or thought representation in the interviews, upon which entire sentences or multiple sentences were put in quotation marks within interview quotations. However, where we believed ambiguity might arise, we indicated the language as either "[ENG]" or "[CAN]" at the end of such direct speech or thought representation. Since Cantonese pronouns are not gendered in speech, whenever the gender of the person interviewees were referring to was unclear, we defaulted to the use of female pronouns.

To safeguard the anonymity of participants further, specific references to specialties or specialist procedures were deleted, and replaced with generic information placed in square brackets (for instance "[a specialty]" or "[a specialist procedure]"). Not all references to specialties or specialist procedures required such editing: for instance, many specialties have a surgical work component, and there are several types of specialist surgeons apart from general surgeons, so to include the information that a participant conducted surgeries in general was considered non-specific. In addition, for participants to explain that they conducted particular specialist procedures as part of their training as housemen, who generally need to rotate around different specialist units, would be similarly non-specific, so such references were not modified.

The resulting themes emerging from the interview data fell under the following five broad groups. These groups provided additional order to the various themes:

Thematic Groups

1. Doctors' reasons for remaining in public hospital work.
2. Standards of medical work set by doctors.
3. Work problems in public hospitals.
4. Personal problems caused by work.
5. Strategies to cope with work demands.

Only group 1 ("doctors' reasons for remaining in public hospital work") contained further categories for the themes, which helped separate the main reasons doctors discussed:

Doctors' Reasons for Remaining in Public Hospital Work

a. Ideals and meanings in work.
b. Problems in the private sector.
c. Work benefits.

The other four groups did not require such an additional level, instead containing themes directly (Fig. 2.2). As mentioned, the benefit of thematic analysis is that it can help put order to a large amount of interview data, such as in this study, in order to address the research aims. However, the possible drawback is also that this can surrender participants' voices to researchers'. To mitigate this, and to achieve the intended focus in this study on doctors' own expressions of views and experiences, the following section representing the results will quote extensively from the interviews, allowing doctors' to be heard in their own words—although for interviews conducted in Cantonese, these were in translation—and giving these greater immediacy and impact. These direct quotations reveal the spectrum of reflections, experiences, and moments in their work.

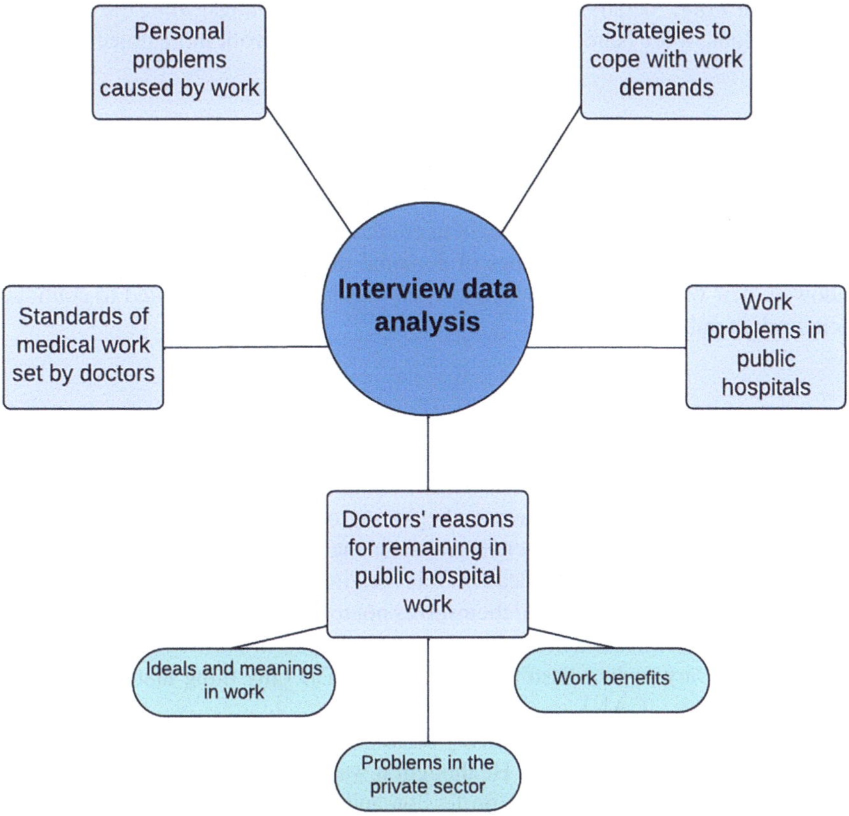

Fig. 2.2 Diagram of the groups and categories that contain interview themes

2.3 Results

2.3.1 Doctors' Reasons for Remaining in Public Hospital Work

This group contains the wide variety of reasons that doctors gave for wanting to remain in the public hospital sector. The first category under this group, "ideals and meanings in work," details more subjective views and meanings, while the other two categories look at the benefits of staying in public sector work more objectively.

2.3.1.1 Ideals and Meanings in Work

This category contains themes that describe doctors' aspiration to higher and more abstract ideals of work that they sought to emulate and live up to. The category also contains themes of additional types of personal meanings and values that doctors endowed their work with, and which created reasons why they wanted to continue their work in public hospitals.

Keeping One's Initial Idealism Close

A number of doctors expressed the usefulness of the idealism with which they viewed the profession prior to and at the very beginning of their journey as doctors. This became an enduring reason for them to remain in the public sector. A common phrase they used to express such initial idealism was "original intention" (「初衷」 or 「初心」), which they used to remind themselves not to lose sight of such idealism. One doctor said: "My original intention has not changed. It's still wanting to help people." He stated that "my 'value' hasn't changed much. The only thing that's changed is the approach I use" [CAN].

A second doctor also said: "I think my original intention has not really changed. If it had, I would have already left." He thought it was important "to 'keep' reminding myself why I originally chose this profession and why I do this, why I work in the public hospital" [CAN]. He elaborated: "I hope that I won't forget why I chose to do this in the first place. I think there are a few things that are very important for being a doctor: you need to have some 'empathy,' and some 'compassion,' which are very important" [CAN]. When asked how he could retain such values, he answered:

> I just do. I just "keep" reminding myself why I started doing this, and how despite the hardship it's worth it, because "at the end of the day," what we want is not some certificate of appreciation—[...] what we want most of all is for patients to get better. "Even" if they can't—because we often see "cancer patients," and we can actually only extend their lives—we hope this extended time means a good "quality of life," and is not one where we just prescribe medications that cause them a lot of suffering, for just some "numerical" "improvement." [CAN]

A third doctor discussed how he reminded trainees of their initial idealism:

> I often ask them [interns] how they responded to the question of why they wanted to be doctors at the medical "school interview[s]." Of course you can say that it was just an "interview," so the "package" [to present oneself with] is always that one wants to help other people. But I think that one must bear responsibility for "adher[ing] to" one's words. I think you must think carefully about why you want to be a doctor. Of course, to be very honest, a doctor's salary is good, benefits are good, and "social status" is high, so you have many "privilege[s]." But I myself also want to remind everyone what their initial goal was at the "interview" stage. You can't forget your original intention. I think that's very important. When I have time, I also remind myself what I thought and said at my "interview." [CAN]

One's original intention becomes a duty to hold oneself to, which creates an additional value to one's work. Although wanting to help others can seem a very unoriginal intention, it can be a powerful one in its very simplicity. As another doctor commented:

> The most clichéd and superficial reason is that you want to help patients. I think right now I'm continuing this [...]: helping patients to improve, that is, giving them treatment so that their bodies and mental state, their "mental health" and their "quality of life," improve. These things I've always wanted to do, or thought that I should do, from the beginning till now. [CAN]

Another doctor said on advice she would give to medical students to help them stay in the public sector:

> I don't know if it applies to them, but just to share what my own "value[s]" are: I think [you should] remember why you chose the profession of being a doctor. [...] When you entered medical school to enter this profession, what was your reason? The reason why I said this doesn't "apply to everyone" is because some people enter [the medical profession] to earn money—although I think this is very unintelligent, because being a doctor does not earn the most money. But I think at the beginning most people are "enthusiastic." My own sense observing "medical student[s]" now is that most are still very passionate. So I think it's very important to carefully think about and remember your original intention, of why you wanted to be a doctor when you first got in. If you hold this reason close to you, then "somehow" it can help you remain in the public sector, because apart from the fact that the "majority" of people are [served by] the public system, if you want to do something very well, then of course you want to help the most people possible, and to help the most people possible, of course [you should be in the] public sector. [...] So this is first: you hold on to the reason why you wanted to be in this line of work.
>
> Second, the typical grand ideals of becoming a doctor: I want to cure patients, and I want to help them escape their dire straits. The people who are truly in dire straits are those who are in the public system. So if you hold on to these most important "value[s]," you will stay here. But also, these things I'm thinking about are a bit idealized. The "value[s]" [that support] remaining in the public sector need such idealization, because to be honest, the public sector is in reality not ideal. Apart from "stability" in work, other things are not ideal. So if you want to stay in an unideal environment, you must have some "higher-end" [values]—we call this the "superego"—some idealized things that can help you stay. [CAN]

Such constant reminding oneself of being a doctor as sustained by ideals made the doctor an active agent in her professional life, rather than a passive receiver of working conditions that could gradually erode the initial passion with which one entered the profession. When she talked about one particular case she handled as a doctor, she commented:

> So you'll feel that you've had an "impact" on their [patients'] lives, that I've left a mark [...] Because of these things, I get the feeling that I've chosen the right subject. I think that when I chose this subject, I hoped to do things that could really change more people's lives." [CAN]

Remembering why she chose this field helped her clearly recognize throughout her career the times when these reasons were realized, creating additional meaning to her work for herself. This can help amplify the positive influence of making a difference, as another doctor expressed when he pushed against resistance to operate on a patient in order to save the patient's life. The moment his patient woke up—recovered—after the surgery made a lasting impact on him: "This 'scenario' was exactly the same as the one I saw four years ago when [my mentor] performed this surgery and the patient suddenly woke up on the operating table. This 'scenario' was my initial reason for wanting to enter [this specialty]" [CAN].

The advice that one doctor would offer medical students was: "When you feel really defeated, when you really want to quit, try to think back to why you chose a specialty in the first place." This is what he would choose to say to them at orientation talks:

> Inevitably, there's a point where you want to quit medical [work]. [...] [J]ust think back to why you got into medical [work]. If you got into medical [work] because of the wrong reasons, then I don't believe you would stay, but if you got into medical [work] because you really want to look after patients, then that's a different story. It will continue to be difficult, but there are moments that you will feel like you've really made a difference. Those are the moments you try to remember and look back to.

The initial reason for entering the profession can then define and give shape to the meaning of one's public hospital medical career.

Most of the doctors quoted above described retaining their initial idealism as a challenge. For them, the fear was that they might lose sight of their initial ideals. As one doctor said: "I do hope that I can keep this 'passion' and not have it disappear" [CAN]. However, not all doctors shared this fear. Another doctor said:

> I've always kind of had the ambition to help people since I was little. Before, when people would talk about what they wanted to do when they were older, if one wanted to help people, these kinds of fields, such as the healthcare field, were very "common." In the end I really chose to enter medicine. [CAN]

She thought that "my overall direction hasn't really changed. I'm still full of enthusiasm. Before, when I started work, I wanted to help people. Now I also want to help people" [CAN].

Non-Materialist Thinking

A non-materialist way of thinking undergirded some of the quotations under the previous theme, where instead of focusing on the money to be earned from their profession, doctors instead focused on an idealism that was not connected to monetary concerns. This theme of "non-materialist thinking" was created to express interviewees' direct and explicit views on money, although such views were of course intricately intertwined with their other views on the value of work.

Several doctors mentioned that earning money was, to them, not the primary driver, although they were very aware of being able to earn more in the private sector. These doctors' philosophy regarding money was such that they did not mind earning less if they could find personal sources of meaning in their public sector hospital work, and if their income was sufficient for their needs. One doctor said:

> [My specialty] earns the most money [in the private sector]. But money, for me, has never been the thing that has most attracted me. My religion—I'm a "Christian"—[means] my aim has never been about how much I can gain, but how much I can help others. So perhaps the positioning of my "value" is already different. "Instead of" looking at how much […] I can earn or get, I put more emphasis on how I can help others and have the biggest impact if I "stay" in my "position." If I were in the "private" sector, I would earn a lot more money, maybe 10 times or even 20 times, especially [in] [my specialty]. But you would only see "low-risk cases." [CAN]

Such personal philosophy could also be influenced by their upbringing. Another doctor said:

> When I was little, the way I was brought up was very "typical." We lived in public housing and my family was very poor. I think having enough money is already "okay." Some people who have gone into private practice earn a lot of money. Of course not everyone does, but some earn a bit more. But I think money is not the most important thing. [CAN]

A third doctor also said:

> When I was little, I had a very simple way of looking at doctors, which is that they help people. Those who want to earn money have left [the public sector] already. Helping people is the number one priority. The moment it gets busy, you realize this immediately. I think "at the end of the day," it's just the same line: an emphasis on helping people. [CAN]

He thought that "I don't need to go out and make money" [CAN]. A fourth doctor's view was in agreement with this: "To be very honest, the salary is not particularly high. Those who want to earn money have gone into the 'private' sector already" [CAN].

Not being primarily motivated by money could also be due to doctors not having pressing financial needs. One doctor said: "I don't have financial or family needs that would compel me to immediately go out into the 'private' sector. So why don't I stay here for the time being? And the work is stable" [CAN]. A second doctor said: "I think I have the luxury of not having […] the financial pressure that some people do." A third doctor said: "In terms of living, my requirements are relatively basic. I don't really mind if I don't earn that much money" [CAN]. A fourth doctor said: "Our demands are modest, and our 'financial burden' is not very big. So I think 'monetary gain' is not what I want" [CAN]. He thought that "the more power you have, the bigger of course your 'responsibility' is":

> Some people think it's very heroic work. But I myself don't think God wants you to be a hero. If God gave you the ability to be a doctor, you have to make good use of this ability to help people in need, "rather than" moving to the private sector to earn big money. I'm not "pinpoint[ing]" [blame onto] my classmates in the private sector, but I myself think that the need in the public sector is very large. [CAN]

Another doctor elaborated on how securely her identity was founded on the work she did, instead of material trappings being necessary for bolstering her confidence levels. She said: "I don't very much like or yearn for that sort of 'luxurious lifestyle.' If I did, I wouldn't have become a [specific medical specialist]" [CAN]. She viewed her "material wants [as] relatively small. [...] I carry a $20 bag to work, though sometimes I do think about whether that's a bit too 'cheap'" [CAN]. This professional self-confidence meant that she thought:

> I'm relatively fulfilled inside. I don't need something external to increase my confidence levels. Maybe my work ability has already been affirmed by "patients": "patient's feedback" has allowed me to discover when what I say, and using what "EQ," leads to all of them saying they want me to keep seeing them. So I already receive a sense of fulfilment in this regard, and I don't need to seek this externally. I don't need to depend on flashy cars or brand-name handbags. So yes, I think that right now I'm situated in a state of confidence, which is quite special. I have never before been so confident. I don't [work] for personal gain, [...] for an individual sense of superiority or for an individual sense of achievement. [CAN]

This effacement of her ego despite her increase in self-confidence became greater the more she advanced in her career:

> When starting work, your value system may not be entirely clear. Sometimes you think, your attire can't look too ugly, or else people will look down on you. Or you secretly think that in the workplace there are people who will treat you better because they think you have money, and worse if they think you are poor. So now I've reached a state where I couldn't care less about whether you think I have money or not. I wear what I'm comfortable in. I "respect" my own "profession" as a doctor. [CAN]

Work as a Higher Calling

Quotations under this theme shared one common trait: their characterization of the profession as a "calling" (the actual English word doctors used in Cantonese interviews), "mission," or personal "dedication." This could be in a secular sense, which in turn derived from the original sense of the word "profession" as a religious calling. It could also be a religious value to doctors, so that their work was what they felt they had been called to by a higher spiritual power.

Although there are some overlaps between this theme and the two previous themes, quotations here ultimately point towards the idea of work as a higher calling. For instance, one interviewee started off by explaining how some doctors could be driven by an extreme desire for money, and then juxtaposed this with his ideal of his work as a "calling," saying:

> I think Hong Kong is very "outcome-oriented." Studying is for exams, exams are for getting high grades, and high grades are to enter university. Each thing has a purpose. For them,

> coming here to receive training, all they want is to get that "certificate," [...] so that they can become a private doctor with [...] a monthly salary of a million dollars. Then they can enjoy the life they want, including eating good stuff, living in a very big house, having 30 dogs, hiring 40 domestic helpers. They have their "utopia." Not every doctor treats being a doctor as their "calling." Maybe it's a stepping stone so that they can get the life they want out there. But there's no right or wrong. It's just that each person's choices are different. [CAN]

A second doctor said: "I think [...] for doctors in general, we don't think of [our work] as a 'job.' Although it's a 'professional job,' it is in fact a 'calling.' You should really feel that you have a 'mission' to help 'patients.' And not just 'patients,' but also their 'family' [CAN]."

A third doctor did not use the word "calling," but conveyed this meaning by describing his work as a personal dedication in a religious sense. He said:

> I used to read a lot of biographies, and I'd choose a lot of biographies by Chinese and Western medicine doctors. Before, I watched a [...] Korean drama series about a male doctor named Hui Jun. I think that series had a big "impact" on me, allowing me to believe that I can "sacrifice" or dedicate my life to this line of work. [In addition,] there is my religion. I'm a "Christian," and I think helping others is part of the natural order. Before I entered the field, I vividly remember there was a pastor [...] who told me that patients put their lives in your hands, that is, not just to treat their illnesses, but to treat them holistically, to treat their lives. Even now, I think these words really touched me, and they often come back in my mind. Therefore, I think: "Yes, I've been in this field for 10 years, and of course my dedication can't be at this high point every day—there are highs and lows. But I will persist. I will not carelessly and perfunctorily see a 'patient.' I will continue in the public system, and do the best I can. [CAN]

A fourth doctor similarly tied the meaning of his work to his religion, saying:

> I have religious faith. [...] I believe in God. [...] I think about the meaning of my life, and the meaning of my work. Of course when you're at a low point in life, you'll think that thinking about these things is a bit useless. But I often think about why God placed me in this work. [CAN]

Other doctors, although not seeing their work through a religious lens, conveyed the secular sense of their work as embodying higher level purpose. One doctor said: "I think most doctors still stay in the public system because they have this sense of mission or [. . .] fulfilment." Another doctor also used the English word "mission": "My confidence is something that being a doctor has given me. I think this work has led me to attain my life's meaning, that is, I think this job is the most suitable one for me. Maybe it's a 'mission' [CAN]." A third doctor said: "I've never expected to have 'work-life balance,' because I don't 'treat' being a doctor as a 'job.' I really treat it as a 'career.' [...] When you hand a patient over to me, or when a patient seeks me out, I want to do my best, to do everything well" [CAN]. Although he used the English word "career" here in an otherwise Cantonese interview, the way in which he distinguished it from the English word "job" again indicated that he looked beyond the work as merely a wage-earning job, endowing it with a sense of higher meaning in the relationship between himself and his work.

Fulfilment from Helping Patients

Under this theme that is very much in line with common expectations of the meaning of doctors' work, interviewees mainly described their love of helping patients in times of need. More noteworthy here are the ways in which doctors frequently described such personal satisfaction: as hinging on their work being in the public sector, and in relation to the challenging work conditions here.

One doctor said: "Sometimes, in that moment of being able to help patients, you will think that not sleeping for 40 hours was worth it." A second doctor explained:

> To be able to keep doing this is not hardship. In fact, I think it's the opposite. I think that being able to help patients makes me very happy. This feeling is very precious. [...] I think what I do is meaningful. Because of this meaning, I will continue to do what I'm doing. [CAN]

A third doctor recounted his joy in seeing his patient's rapid recovery, which was "unexpected" [ENG], and said that such cases "give me the power to continue my work, although it's really tough working here in the public sector, and you are faced with lots of 'demand[s]'" [CAN]. A fourth doctor explained how he wished to stay in the public sector because of wanting to help patients in a practical way:

> The history of medicine is that we were just some wise old man or woman in the village or in a township somewhere, who just happened to know a few tricks up his sleeve of how to cure trauma wounds, for example, or how to make a person feel comfortable when they had undeniably unsalvageable conditions [...]. At that time, they would pay visits to [...] that patient's family and to their home. Why did our profession have to be put on a pedestal? Yeah, that's why I wouldn't want to go to the private sector.

A fifth doctor described helping patients as her primary source of meaning:

> The 'satisfaction' from being a doctor, do you think it comes from 'admin[istrative]' [work]? Of course it comes from patients. Therefore, very often, it makes you very happy to see patients, especially patients whom you have been able to help. In fact, when you see patients getting better, it makes you happy. [CAN]

Not all cases doctors handle have good outcomes, and not all patients are grateful for doctors' help, but the cases with positive outcomes, one doctor explained, kept him going. He said:

> There are one or two "negative cases" [with negative outcomes] each year that leave a deep impact. But most [cases], that is 99%, don't have problems. But the "cases" that make you unhappy will cause you to be "down" for a period of time. But [...] ultimately most "case[s]" are very good, and many very ill patients [...] recover, and can go out and continue to *yum cha*. If you didn't treat them, they might have already died, and wouldn't be able to play with their grandchildren. We have helped many such patients. [CAN]

Thus he thought that "having learned this [specialist] procedure, being able to help people, and having a sense of achievement can 'keep' me working here. In one year I have been able to help many such patients. This is very meaningful" [CAN]. Another doctor said: "Perhaps it's just 'one out of 100' who will genuinely thank you. But I feel I can help many people. I genuinely feel that even if they're not very 'grateful,' I have helped them" [CAN].

Doctors' work often became turning points in patients' lives. Talking of a case when he was able to make a huge difference to a patient, another doctor said: "This is not able to be weighed in terms of money. It was something that relied on my own pair of hands and what I studied, and then being able to help someone. This is extraordinary" [CAN]. Another doctor described turning a case that others had given up on entirely and miraculously around for the better, giving her a deep sense of fulfilment from her work:

> The more you learn, the more you know. When you have people supporting you, when you have a whole team there to support you, you will find that it's 'amazing': life can be less easily lost. It turns out that when others have given [a case] up for dead, they can in fact 'survive.' [...] So I think it's really meaningful. [CAN]

She told the interviewer that "I hope that through what you write, we can let more people know that in fact in public hospitals there are still many doctors whose hearts are dedicated to helping our 'patients'" [CAN].

Other doctors emphasized their relationship with patients and their family as a source of fulfilment. One doctor said:

Every day, when I see them very happy that [the patients] can be discharged from the hospital, their "grateful[ness]," I feel I have given hope to the family. That's why I still like my line of work. I feel my "specialty" is a happy one. [CAN]

She described her first exposure to her specialty as something joyful: "I suddenly felt, 'wow, I feel very happy, the whole ward is very happy.' And I felt that the family was very 'hopeful' when I could help them. So I suddenly wanted to stay here" [CAN]. Another doctor similarly saw her work as spreading joy to many others: "I feel that on a certain level I'm benefiting others. I have the sense that I'm sharing [...]. I hope to be able to share happiness, share positive energy, share 'kindness.' So this job is not just for my personal gain" [CAN]. A third doctor said:

> From when they [patients] see me for the first time, to when I start doing investigations, perform surgery, and then have follow-up consultations with them every one to two years—every time we see each other, the feeling is like seeing family again. Although this is [built up] little by little, the feeling is good. If you ask me, I quite like this kind of relationship. [CAN]

A fourth doctor commented:

> Actually the "workload" is heavy, and you'll be under "pressure." But at the same time, if you really care about your "patient[s]," and you really treat your "case[s]" seriously, then you get a lot of "satisfaction," because when you see them get better after surgery, or the "patient" comes back and is very "grateful" towards you, this gives you a lot of "satisfaction", and "this is also something that keeps me doing" [ENG]. [CAN]

A fifth doctor was unfazed by the heavy time demand of the many consultations. He said:

> I love holding medical consultations. I love communicating with patients. Some doctors think giving medical consultations is too much trouble, that there are many cases, and

> that it's suffering. But I think it's nothing much. I quite enjoy communicating with family members. If I can teach them something, simple things that they can learn to handle, I feel very happy. So I enjoy this, and I keep going. [CAN]

He added that "the patients I treated when I first entered the profession […] have grown up. I'm still in touch with some of them. Seeing them all grown up and healthy makes me think that the things I did before were very meaningful" [CAN].

Finally, one doctor discussed the opportunities he had in the public hospital setting to continue his learning even after attaining his specialist status, to the extent where he gained specialist status in a second field. Although parts of the following quotation could also be categorized under the later theme entitled "further training and enhanced learning," the interviewee's overriding reason was to fulfil his drive to help patients, as he explained:

> Staying here with the "HA," […] you can just "clock in" and "clock out," and have standard working hours, and that's it. But that's very boring. I am relatively "curious and inquisitive," and I like to "keep" some things novel, to "keep" on learning things, learning "skills." Very often, at public hospitals, or at least university hospitals, there's a much greater chance of having those "opportunities." If you go out into the private sector, you have much fewer of these. For example, if you are out in the private sector, you're earning money, and you wouldn't suddenly study one more "specialty" [which is what he did].
>
> You asked me just now why I did this. […] The "patient" is "mainly" the reason. We take care of many "patient[s]" in [a particular specialist unit], but in a very "fragmented" way. Perhaps we make the diagnosis at the beginning, and then it's as if we throw them to another department, and then they come back in the end. I think [. .] that's not particularly comprehensive from a "patient journey" perspective. The "patient" wouldn't feel very good about this, because everyone is only concerned with their own area.
>
> So my reasoning is that I want to learn more, learn in a more complete way to help patients. […] Passing the exams of one more "fellowship" was therefore "mainly" driven by our daily interaction with them, and feeling sorry for "patient[s]." There was a "need," a "niche," and a "service gap." I thought that after doing this, […] even if you say that there is no other "outcome," then at least it can lead to them feeling that there is someone who is there from the beginning to the end to take care of them, to watch over them, instead of them being tossed back and forth. […] Because within the "HA," what tends to happen is that when people ask things, they will answer: "This doesn't have to do with me—ask the neighboring specialty." [CAN]

Seeing such patients' concerns from the perspective of his different specialty helped him understand that patients' emotional and informational needs could remain seriously unmet by the care of the main specialty handling their case, leading to his desire and drive to help them:

> I think sometimes from an observer's perspective, you can see things more clearly. So I thought, why not study [this additional specialty] as well? Then [our care] can be more comprehensive. […] Especially for patients who are young when they become ill, very often they have other psychosocial issues, some have fertility issues, some have counselling issues because their family are there with them. Very often our care is not adequate, because within the Hospital Authority or even in the private sector, there are no people who specialize in helping these types of patients. I myself have this interest, and I think I have this ability to help them. [CAN]

Duty to Patients and Society

Alongside gaining a sense of personal satisfaction from being able to help patients, doctors also felt the obligation—including a moral obligation—to help patients. Several doctors spoke about this sense of duty in terms of repaying a debt they thought they had incurred due to having been supported by society throughout their education and training as medical doctors. One doctor said:

> I come from a very poor family. But I applied for whatever subsidy I could. I remember we had very little money to spend towards my studies. We paid for kindergarten out of our own money, but after kindergarten we got money from the government. At university I got "grants" and "loans." So basically, my entire learning and study journey, and strictly speaking the "degree" I obtained, was paid for by "taxpayers." So I've always thought that it was because of taxpayers that I was able to obtain my "degree." [...] Our salaries are also high, and this money in fact also comes from "taxpayers." And the taxpayers from when I was little are now all "elderly"—perhaps they're all retired. Those retired people very often cannot afford to go "private," because they don't have money. So they end up in the public system as part of the "aging population." So sometimes, when I see that "population," I think: these people paid for my education when I was young, paid for my tuition fees perhaps. [CAN].

When she went overseas for further training, she again thought about the obligation she owed to repay this to society:

> I took a "break" and studied in the UK for a year. I left the "HA" at the time. I got a Hong Kong "scholarship" to go there. Ultimately, that "scholarship" was paid for by the government. So I [...] made a "promise" at the time I got the scholarship that upon my return from learning, I would contribute back to Hong Kong society, this "system." To be involved in a "system" and establish a "service," you wouldn't go to the private sector. Although my ability upon returning has not been enough to establish a "service," at the very least I think that it's better that after learning some "skills," I serve the "majority" of the "population." So for this reason I've stayed in the public sector. [CAN]

Another doctor similarly thought that "I feel, especially if you studied in Hong Kong, in a way, your school fees have been subsidized by the government." A third doctor thought:

> No matter how bad the public sector is, on some level it has trained me up. I won't speak for others, but my feeling is that I want to contribute back to this place, if I see that this place has a need. But of course, I don't have financial burdens at the moment, so I can say this relatively easily. [CAN]

A fourth doctor expressed her disappointment at younger colleagues leaving soon after completing their training:

> Many people leave after they've finished "train[ing]." It is really disappointing to us. From the perspective of a "team," of course if you lose a colleague, the dullest way of expressing this is that you lose one pair of hands: "Do you want to work us to death?" [...] But in fact I think there's something else that leads to me feeling very disappointed. [...] I'm very grateful I have a group of very good "senior[s]" who gave us a lot of care and knowledge and time to nurture you, to teach you. You really "work as a team," and you really work and strive hard together. [...] But why when everyone spent so much effort to nurture you, do you just leave with a swish? I myself can't really accept this. Of course I'm not "comment[ing]" that they're definitely wrong in doing this, because they have many other "consideration[s]"—perhaps

> "family issues," because at public hospitals [...] we need to take care of many things at the same time, and you really need to be prepared for 24/7 work. I could at midnight have to return to hospital to handle something that other people can't handle. [...] It is without doubt very "stressful" and very exhausting [work], but it's something "meaningful." [CAN]

There were other reasons behind interviewees' deep sense of obligation and responsibility to genuinely help patients. For one doctor, his religion played a key role:

> You can see [patients] in a perfunctory way. Maybe you give them a "follow-up," or you just do "procedure[s]" in a relatively careless way. You may be able to get past yourself, you may be able to get your salary, and you may be able to get off work at 5:30 pm, but I think your "impact" on their lives is actually larger than you may imagine. Every time I reach this point in my thinking, I get very scared. I feel that I do not want to have a "negative impact" on a "patient," that is, my own feeling is that God does not want me to be a doctor in this way. [CAN]

Another doctor thought that he owed patients and the community a duty to provide good service: "90% of the patients in Hong Kong attend a public hospital, and I don't want it to fail. I think it's a bit of giving back to the community as well." He added: "I've regularly thought about quitting the public sector [...]. But on the other hand, there are patients that I have good rapport with, right? That's one thing: my patients." This sense of responsibility then provided a connection to the public system that he did not wish to break.

Feeling Indispensable

Unlike the previous theme, this theme focuses primarily on interviewees' sense of being absolutely—perhaps even desperately—needed in the public system, rather than solely on contributing to society and helping patients, although these may form part of interviewees' motivation expressed in this theme as well. They show how the value of doctors' skills interpellates[1] or hails the doctors, creating a strong tie to the public system in which they work.

This could be due to the shortage of specialists or skills in the public sector, or due to the demand for public sector healthcare in Hong Kong. For instance, one doctor said:

> In our hospital, there are only two or three people who possess [these specialist] skills. If I leave, then in the whole of [this hospital district] [...] there will only be one person who could perform this kind of surgery. That would be very bad. I think that having learned this, being able to help people, and having a sense of achievement, can "keep" me here to do my work. [CAN]

Another doctor said that the type of surgery she could do was "a specialist interest. Very few people in Hong Kong, or even in South-East Asia, can perform this surgery" [CAN]. A third doctor thought:

---

[1] Here we borrow the surface meaning of this term used by the philosopher Louis Althusser without making full use of his idea of subject-constitution within social structures.

> You feel exhausted, but there's a patient who needs your help, and on that day, in the whole of the [district], there's only you who can help them. If they don't get help, [...] if they don't undergo surgery, their mortality rate is 70% [...]. And that night only you can help them. Then actually, when you successfully do the surgery, your sense of fulfilment is huge. I think that's what some people describe as very much enjoying the "need to be needed." When you manage to help them, to help the family, when the whole family thanks you, that feeling can "overcome" all the negativity that has gone before. [CAN]

This sense of being absolutely needed amplified the sense of fulfilment derived from work: "I've grown up, and 'acquire[d]' some skills, some things that only specialists can do. You think, 'What I can do in fact very few people can do.' At the same time, the patient needs this service. Then you feel a sense of fulfilment" [CAN]. A fourth doctor said:

> Outside [the public hospital system] there are no "ICU unit[s]" to "support" this [patient group]. They are all referred to public hospitals. So I think my value lies in being a "gate-keeper." [...] The reason why I like being here is because I think what the outside cannot do doesn't matter for patients, because they can come to the public hospital and I can still help them no matter what. [CAN]

She also thought that "being a 'gatekeeper' involves my ego just a tiny little bit. Others cannot help them but I can, doing just my little bit" [CAN]. A fifth doctor said:

> At the time, I was a student, and I knew nothing. But [the patient] then said that she had to undergo this surgery [to get better]. "My child is still so young. I need to do this no matter what." And in this world no one could help her but [a specific medical specialty]. Not only that, but only university hospitals had the technology to do this. So I thought, wow [...]. It turns out that studying so much means that you really become the only person in this world able to help this patient. What she said had a huge impact on me. [CAN]

A sixth doctor said:

> Perhaps you have heard of reports saying that public hospitals cover 90% of patients, and private hospitals 10%. But the ratio of doctors is half to half. So I'm inclined towards staying in the public system to help these people. [...] I'm not trying to discredit the "private" sector, but at least my "calling"... my feeling is that the public system needs me more. That's why I'll stay. [CAN]

Even when doctors were off work they may feel that they were so needed that they voluntarily opted to perform work duties. One doctor said:

> When I'm off work I also need to reply to these "message[s]" [from work], but I'm happy to, because I don't want to delay things for patients. Or maybe sometimes I know that another colleague is up to their eyeballs in work, and is seeing patients without even having had a meal. [CAN]

Not responding makes her "feel unsettled. It's a 'moral obligation' [CAN].

Finding Work Intrinsically Meaningful

The expressions of the intrinsic meaning of work under this theme include quotations in which the meaning of work was described as an inward movement towards the self, as opposed to an outward movement from work towards the more social, moral, and instrumental functions it could serve, which have been covered in some of the themes discussed so far. This is not to draw a hard-and-fast distinction between the personal and other domains, such as the social, which would be impossible. Rather, this separate theme includes quotations where the emphasis is relatively more on the self than on these other domains.

One doctor spoke of the intrinsic enjoyment he felt doing his work, with minimal reference to other reasons in that instance in the interview. He said:

> Because I really enjoy my work, I don't think it's a "burden." Of course I have had to sacrifice some things, for example time with my family, or a slightly worse relationship with my family. But this is my interest. I don't treat it as work, because daily work is my interest, not a task. "Whenever I go to work it's exhausting": I don't ever think like this. [...] Right now, when I have to do a bit more, for instance see [patients'] family for longer, or taking a longer time to handle things, all these things make up the meaning of my work. I don't think of it as a "task." [CAN]

He thought that "Ultimately, if you don't 'enjoy' your work, it will become exhausting" [CAN].

Another doctor expressed the intrinsic meaning of her work to her in terms of a sense of innate fit between herself and her work. She said:

> It's not about "work-life balance." My latest thought is that it's "work-health balance," because when I engage myself in work, work is "part of" my "life." Actually when I do my work well, I can perhaps "fulfil" my "purpose" in life. I "enjoy" it, so it's not that I only become happy after I get off work. [...] When work gets busy, perhaps my "EQ" will become lower, but when I'm at the level where I can "handle" it, then "most of the time" I'm in fact in a state where I feel that going to work is very fulfilling, full of learning opportunities. [CAN]

She indicated that she was the author of the meaning of her work, which spoke to and taught her as a person, and shaped and enhanced her moral values:

> My goals in life, and how they can be expressed in this work, make me think this job suits me. For instance, after coming into contact with many people and things, and after all my life experiences at this age, I think that "kindness" is more important than intellect. All these years, in my work, I have repeatedly learned this. The things that I myself throw out there are "positivity" and "kindness," and I also receive some "positivity" and "kindness" [in return]. This makes me feel relatively fulfilled. So perhaps I myself am endowing my work with meaning, that is, I am the lead I think that if my work is to have meaning, I have to become this type of doctor. [CAN]

Therefore, she did not "get upset just because I need to handle work-related things in my off time" [CAN]. Because of the aptness of her work, which made her feel "fulfilled in my life," she also did not "draw a strict line between work and recreation. This is because when I'm really engaged in my work, and I'm happy doing it, my mood levels can already be very high" [CAN].

Although she said that "in a nutshell, I love this job" [CAN], the workload in the public system could still feel overwhelming at times, so that she "always [thought] that being a 'part-time' public doctor is the happiest thing. The 'nature' of the work would [still be] that of being a public doctor, possessing everything I've said about the richness of 'interactions' with patients, about the content. Life would be very enriched" [CAN]. She gave advice based on her own sense of deep personal belonging to her work:

> If you ask some beginners, that is fresh graduates, to explore which job has meaning, they don't even know the meaning of their own lives, so how can they know which job has meaning? Therefore, maybe they need to find their own bearings, their own "personality trait[s]," what they like. When they go look for a job, that job can "exercise" and "execute" these "personality traits." Only then can they be engaged. [CAN]

We see in these quotations how work had become not only part of life for her, but how work was seen *as* life, instead of compartmentalized within it.

Patients from All Walks of Life

As the Introduction and some interviewees already mentioned, the public hospital system serves the vast majority of patients in Hong Kong, not only because of the nominal cost to patients, but also because the private system can and does refuse treatment to patients with complex conditions, sending them to public hospitals instead. This theme shows how public hospital doctors thought it was important that they could help patients in need who might otherwise not be able to afford private healthcare, or who might be refused treatment there. Although there is some overlap with other themes, in particular "fulfilment from helping patients," the defining focus here is on the sheer scope of patients who could be cared for.

Numerous doctors mentioned how meaningful it was to them to be able to treat less privileged patients. One interviewee said:

> People who have an illness want the opportunity to receive treatment. "I think that's the role for us in the public hospital" [ENG]. We don't get to choose: we must "treat" every person who is referred to us. Only then can we "treat" them "to the best of our abilities." [...] I think this is something very meaningful [...]. For instance, a while ago, perhaps because of "COVID," many people who had fever went to private hospitals, and were denied entry, with them saying that if you had a fever, we wouldn't see you. You're a hospital, yet you say that you won't see anyone with a fever. It's difficult to imagine that something like that can be said. [...] I myself am very "against" this, so being a public hospital doctor is something I'm very proud of. [CAN]

Another doctor said: "One or two 'case[s]' left an impression on me, because [...] they were Comprehensive Social Security Assistance recipients, and didn't have much money. If they couldn't afford to see private doctors, [...] then where would they end up?" [CAN]. A third doctor said that despite difficulties at work, he found joy in the thought of being able to help all patients:

> There was a time when I found it very exhausting. [...] Before, I would of course mind it when patients, after surgery... that is, why would there be people complaining that you caused bruises or pain? [...] But sometimes I think, the ones with money go to private hospitals, but it's sad for the ones without any choice. We can help these people who are less "wealthy." I'm happy about this. [CAN]

He elaborated on this feeling:

> I think money is not really the most important thing. In contrast, I think the sense of achievement from being able to handle complex "case[s]"—when you can help some really critical patients, and they can go home after surgery—makes me really happy. Although they might not thank you, I feel very happy inside. [CAN]

A third doctor said:

> Serving people from grassroots communities to the middle class was an important reason why I entered this profession. I'm not saying that I wouldn't be able to "serve" these people in the "private" sector, but I think at this moment, the "need" in public-sector organizations is huge. This is because in fact doctors or other medical resources are not "equal[ly]" distributed in Hong Kong. [CAN]

A fourth doctor's views were similar:

> Before, when the "technology" [used for certain specialist procedures] was not so common, what perhaps only private hospitals could do would cost a lot. For instance, if I performed [a specialist procedure] at night, perhaps some [private hospitals] would be charging $800,000 to a million. But in some low-income families, many are "breadwinner[s]," and if they really do have [a particular illness], they also need... their need is perhaps even bigger, because they don't have money. If they do have [a particular illness], no one treats them, and they are [incapacitated], it's really tough for the "family." So if there is a "platform" to bring the best medical care to them, to patients in the most need and unable to pay, then this "practice" is very important. [CAN]

A fifth doctor commented: "Ultimately, I want to do things to help people at the grassroots level, or do things that help 'patients'" [CAN].

The huge number and wide variety of patients doctors served then became a reason for, instead of against, staying in public hospitals. One doctor said:

> It's very idealistic, and it's a bit like fighting the strong and helping the weak. I need to help poorer people. Right now I'm not the wealthiest, but I must do this. [...] Amongst doctors, I may not be one who earns a lot of money, and this may not be the place with the most staff. But I'm helping the public. I'm not a very "resourceful" doctor compared to a private doctor, but [...] I'm "serv[ing]" the "majority of" Hong Kongers, the "majority of" the "population." [CAN]

A second doctor said: "I think the benefit of being a doctor is that it's relatively easy to find the meaning of your work. When at a public hospital, you really witness just how many people need care, and your assistance is quite direct." [CAN]. A fourth doctor described how interesting her work was as a result of the number of patients: "Within one day, you can witness the whole spectrum of life. Very wealthy people will come to see doctors, and very poor people will also come to the public hospital to see doctors" [CAN]. Because of this, "the variation in patients is bigger. The most troublesome, the most critical, the most complex. The things that are the most difficult to handle. These will all appear in hospitals. So the 'range' is bigger. All these things are very meaningful" [CAN].

Instigating Social Change

Although treating patients can be seen as a clear social benefit that doctors' work yields, two doctors in this study spoke more explicitly about contributions to society they wished to make, motivated primarily by a desire for social change rather than as starting from a sense of duty, as was the case for quotations included under the theme "duty to patients and society." One doctor saw her role as spreading happiness in society from the simple base of the medical consultation:

> I hope that I can make a positive difference to "interaction[s]" [between people] in this society, making them happy "from" a simple "interaction" inside a small "consultation room." At the same time I'm happy too. So I think that because of this, I'm able to be engaged in this job." [CAN]

Another doctor saw his work as a stepping stone to wider improvements he could make on a societal level:

> I hope that I can make an impact through social change in my position right now. Virchow, a very famous professor of medicine, [of] pathology [...], at the turn of nineteenth century I believe, said that the ills of society are manifested in the ills of the individual patient, and so I take that to heart. [...] I'll take it one step further and say that a lot of the patients we see in a public hospital setting are a direct manifestation of the failures of society. And so, for example, most of our patients come from relatively poor areas in Hong Kong [...] where there are a lot of people that are homeless, drug addicts, people from a lower socioeconomic status. And to see them coming in with [a particular specialist disease], for example, is a prime example of how poor diet, smoking, and drinking contribute to this ultimately catastrophic outcome. And that is where society pays, because taking care of a [...] patient [with a specific disease], especially the ones that we operate on [...], is very resource intensive.

He was now at a stage in his career where he could question his role, and what larger social contributions he could make, more deeply:

> I feel that I might be able to make a change at the at the more fundamental levels in the community. [...] So it's changed quite a bit from just being focused on the task at hand and being focused on the patients, [...] on getting the patient better and looking forward to the next patient, [to] now, in this phase, [...] where I feel that I can avoid seeing these patients [because disease has been prevented] by trying to make a contribution to their welfare at the social level.

He thought that "there are a lot of doctors out there [who,] when they reach a certain point in their career, they feel that they can make an even greater impact," and asked: "So how do you do that? The change you want to enact in the community: what kinds of things do you do? Do you do outreach activities?" He listed some of the many activities he was involved in, such as "trying to inspire the next generation of high school students, or students that are in med school, to get involved in [his specialty]," giving "public talks," "making surgical policy changes in the profession," "working with quite a few NGOs in Hong Kong" to, for example, "engage patients into having better living—mindfulness, dietary adjustments, and so forth," working with the government on a "big data project where we'd like to see if we can identify patients who have no illness whatsoever, no symptoms, [...] [and] predict their risk of [various diseases], [...] [and] intervening earlier," and "working with some [...] private donors [...]—they're from the land development companies here—to see whether or not we can offer [...] halfway houses or beds for people that [...] are physically fit to be discharged, but where the community hasn't had any long-term plan long term institutional care beds yet." In working on all these activities, he used his profession as a platform for social improvement, rather than treating it as defining the limits of what he could do.

Teaching the Next Generation of Doctors

One distinction between public and private sector work that many doctors mentioned was that they could help train the next generation of doctors in the public system. As one doctor put it, "I feel like here [in the public system] you can offer a bit more guidance because there are more juniors under you, [whereas] in private [care] it's just you." Doctors thought of this as beneficial not just to the trainees, but also to themselves and to the work in public hospitals in a variety of ways. For instance, one doctor said: "My current 'team head' [...] always says that when you teach, both the teacher and the student gain something on an 'academic' level. That is, when I teach someone else, I myself can come up with a lot of things" [CAN]. Another doctor said:

> I think after I passed my specialist qualification [exams], in the two to three years after that, because I didn't have any more exam pressure, [...] I learned more things myself, [...] [and] I would think about how to teach others these things. How do I share what I have learned, or lessons learned from mistakes I made, with some "trainees," or other people such as nurses, occupational therapists, and other colleagues I work with? This is also a type of learning: how to share my knowledge, and at the same time within this exchange, I can also learn something, because people looking at things from different angles will sometimes see things differently from me. [CAN]

This was not only edifying to the interviewee, but also enjoyable:

> I like "teaching" others, and this is something that there is much less of in the private sector. [...] It's not just that after I finish a textbook, I'll know how to do something, or how to "translate" that "knowledge" to my "practice." [...] At the beginning [junior colleagues] don't really know how to do it, but then they try to use your method, and slowly discover their own method. If I go to the private sector, I would lose this. [...] When you see them improve, it's something very "rewarding," I think. So this is something that up until now I haven't really wanted to give up. [CAN]

Other doctors saw passing on the baton as their responsibility to the continuity of the system and of the community of doctors. One doctor said: "In the past 10 years or so, my 'role' has been to help 'junior specialist[s]' to build up their 'expertise.'

My 'role' has been that of a 'trainer,' and to help them grow, and to pass on [my knowledge], because I need to retire, right?" [CAN]. Another doctor also thought: "I need to use what I learned before or what I did wrong to teach [trainees]. I think this is a kind of transmission of knowledge, one more thing that is not just for myself" [CAN]. A third doctor said: "Right now I really want to teach my skills to the next generation of [specialist doctors] so that they can help patients. And for this, again, 'team spirit' is very important" [CAN]. A fourth doctor said: "I've suddenly become a 'senior.' Suddenly my 'teaching load' has become heavier. The sense of transmitting knowledge has become bigger. And also, suddenly I feel that I must 'inspire' more than continue to be 'inspire[d]' by my 'senior[s]'" [CAN]. A fifth doctor explained:

> I went from being a "trainee" to being a "supervisor" or "teacher." [...] I don't just teach medical students, but also teach doctors, and even "midwives" [...]. And we also don't just teach the doctors and nurses at our own hospital, but as if we have many tentacles, we also go to many different "conference[s]." So after my roles changed, [...] my "focus" has perhaps also changed. [...] You think about how to "facilitate" "trainee[s]," how to do something well, and how to work as a "team" and maintain our "team spirit." [CAN]

This was one of the reasons why she felt "for the moment, staying at a public hospital, a teaching hospital, means I have a bigger sense of fulfilment" [CAN].

Two doctors emphasized the crucial importance of having mid-level doctors as teachers. One doctor said:

> "Junior[s]" will ask you to help with any questions they have, or with anything they can't handle. The "training" they need as part of their studies and exams is again offered by me. So in fact the middle stratum is a very important stratum. Although being in the middle is very tough, I think being here, I still have a role to play, so I want to do this. Also, I quite like teaching others things, such as skills, all kinds of knowledge, and so on. You don't have this in the private sector. [...] [Here] I can "train" "junior[s]" in the "specialt[ies]" they want to be in. [...] I can teach them how to enter these specialties, and how to deepen their knowledge. I can help them. [CAN]

Another doctor expressed concern that not enough mid-level doctors would stay in the public sector to teach future doctors. She was worried because "you can see that the line of 'succession' will break" [CAN].

Patient Gratitude as Repositories of Value

When patients told doctors how grateful they were to them, doctors tended to remember and hold on to those encounters as repositories of value. One doctor said: "People say you shouldn't derive your own self-worth from external things like [...] people's positive feedback or praise that you get. But [...] it helps, people's appreciation. [...] I think that that's an important thing to keep us going." Another doctor said:

> I have many patients who have followed me for five to 10 years, whom I may have known for over five years from when they first started to become ill till now. Every time they come back they are very "grateful," and they treat me like a "family doctor." It turns out that even in

public hospitals such feelings are still possible. It's very precious. [...] I have my complaints about working at a public hospital, but "at the same time I see the merits of working as a public doctor." [CAN]

A third doctor recounted a time when early in his career a patient's treatment had a poor outcome, and the patient passed away. He said:

Instead of expressing frustration or anger, the son actually told the consultant, thank you for helping my mother. And, you know, from my perspective, it's really extraordinary, because at the end of the day, his mom right died from complications from the surgery. But then the son actually thanked my consultant [the interviewee's superior] because he knew that to begin with, we were trying to save his mother and the consultant basically talked to the patient's son every single day. [...] Even if the worst thing happened, he was still very grateful for what we'd done. These are the moments of satisfaction that I guess doctors really remember for life.

A fourth doctor said: "Sometimes patients remember you, or when they come back, even buy things for you to eat, although of course we can't accept these things. But you will feel happy. They come back and we chat, and it's like seeing an old friend" [CAN].

A fifth doctor focused not on explicit words of gratitude from patients, but on their feedback, which led her to realize the difference she had made to their lives. She said:

Sometimes they will say this [how important she is to the patient] to me, and tell me what I said the last time. It turns out that they take it to heart. Maybe I myself think I'm not saying something in a deliberate way, but they take it very much to heart. [...] So these things "feed back" to me and allow me to see that my every word and every action, my "encounter" with patients, "mean something" to them. [CAN]

She explained that in such moments, "you will feel that you have an 'impact' on their lives. Only because they think you're important will they say these things to you" [CAN]. Despite "getting off work late every day and getting frustrated, I can really 'push' some people to change a bit, and have some 'new insights into life,'" "and this 'feed[s] back' to me that I have some value" [CAN].

2.3.1.2 Problems in the Private Sector

The themes laid out so far have focused on quoting doctors' positive views of their public hospital work, creating reasons to remain in this environment despite some of the drawbacks the interview quotations have already revealed to us. However, doctors also mentioned problems in the private health sector that could negatively impact their medical practice, leading to them being reluctant to join it despite the potentially more lucrative nature of such work.

Commercial Interests

Working in the for-profit private sector may lead to financial concerns influencing the very nature of the work and its priorities, and many interviewees found such a prospect unappealing. One doctor said: "I don't want to go out into the 'private' sector because I don't want something that I like to be tied to money. It's as if the whole thing becomes not 'pure' enough" [CAN]. Another doctor thought:

> "So far" I think I may not be very suited to working in the "private" sector. [...] There are many in the "private" sector who care, and who put their "patient[s]" first. But you would still need to think about a lot more things: money, working with other "agent[s]," and in terms of "treatment" there will be some approaches that are different from those in public hospitals, that is, maybe [...] more "aggressive." [CAN]

A third doctor criticized the private sector in his specialty as consumerist, saying:

> After they see them [doctors] once, and after the surgery is done, then bye bye, they're gone. In fact it's like a shopping experience: [...] I go to a brand name store, I see a pretty handbag, it's what I want, I pay money to buy it, and then I leave. So it's a very "consumer[ist] experience." This is not the kind of doctor-patient "relationship" that I got to know about when I was little. [CAN]

He explained that whereas in the doctor-patient relationship in the public sector, money does not play a role, "in the private sector it's the opposite: everything has to do with money" [CAN]. So "even for something that you may think of as very routine—for instance [a specialist surgery], [which] seems the same everywhere," the actual cost depends on a patient's anatomy, so that "you need to use different equipment," and because of this, "the cost in fact should also be different" [CAN]. However, "in the private system, everything is sold as a package" with a fixed price, resulting in "some colleagues very carefully choosing patients they want to treat" [CAN]. He thought that money-making as a goal might even distort medical decisions, leading to "the use of unnecessary treatments to treat some diseases that shouldn't be treated, or don't need to be treated" [CAN]. For instance,

> There may in fact be no disease, but for the sake of [money], [treatment] has been done. And there's no regulation. It's really eye-opening. [...] "I can only feel sad for the patients." If you've been ill, you'll know that you really want a genuine "opinion." That person may not be able to save you, or may not be able to stop the disease, but "at least they tell you something honest," and it's not for their personal gain. But money is something that can turn someone's head. I've seen many patients who have become bankrupt because of these issues. [CAN]

In addition, the focus on making money would make receiving guidance and training from different doctors "very difficult," because "you work from Monday to Saturday, seeing patients, doing surgeries, helping the clinic earn money. So it would be difficult for me to have the chance to have three months, six months, or even a longer 'training' period" [CAN]. Such a commercial environment might also not lead to a lighter patient load than in the public sector:

> It turns out that private clinics may in fact also have a very high patient load. It really depends on how many "patient[s]" the "clinic" arranges to see a particular doctor. That is, some clinics [...] may arrange 20 "patient[s]" within half an hour, and it's not really "up to" the private doctor to decide how much time to spend on "patient[s]." What is the most "likely" reason for this? [It's] because many doctors take part in conglomerate-based operations, since the cost of the "setup" is just too high. So, for instance, buying one diagnostic machine costs one "million," and another diagnostic machine is one "million," so if you are a "solo practitioner," it's difficult to buy many machines. [...] So many private doctors work as a "group," and behind this "group" can be doctors or non-doctors who are "manager[s]." These "manager[s]" decide the mode of operation of the clinic. Originally I thought that private doctors have a lot of [...] "freedom," but now I hear my colleagues say that in fact this may not necessarily be the case. [CAN]

Other doctors spoke of the possibility of their own values and motivations being affected by the focus on money-making in the private sector. One doctor said that at times in the private sector, "you do things for 'convenience,' for 'speed,' for many things, for money. Perhaps these are not really the things I want to do" [CAN]. Another doctor said:

> If you go out to the private sector, your "mentality" might change. It does feel a bit like doing business. So perhaps when you write a report you will encourage them to do another scan, or there's a chance that you cause them to have a surgery performed. Your "threshold" to do this is lower. But the "public sector" is very different. You don't want them to continue scans. You don't want them to do unnecessary "surger[ies]." So your "threshold of" prescribing these things will be different. I would be a bit concerned myself that, in the "private" sector, I would have these kinds of temptations affecting my "judgement." I don't think this would be very good. [CAN]

A third doctor explained that although work times in the private sector were "more 'flexible,' in fact it's still like a business, that is, it's not as simple as just 'treat[ing] a patient.' There are many things to think about. For instance, you have to think about the 'cost' of 'running your business'" [CAN]. A fourth doctor thought she would not be able to voice her true opinions in the private sector, and that many relationships would become commercial: "If you want to work in the private sector, then you have to keep quiet about some things. [...] The method some people use to do things may not be very appropriate, but [if you are] in the private sector, you don't say anything. [...] You must protect your peers' dignity in the private sector, or their 'brand'" [CAN], so that "the private doctor working alongside you in the private sector [is] like a business partner" [CAN]. Although in the public sector, "you can't directly criticize the department next door either," "the 'degree' is not the same: there is a bigger 'allowance' in public hospitals, and you can communicate more clearly with patients" [CAN]. In addition, "in the private sector, I believe that the doctor-patient relationship is more complicated: [...] the patient has given money to a private doctor, and their expectations are definitely higher. If you say anything amiss, then they can 'badmouth' you and influence your 'career,' and this to some extent will influence the trust that subsequent patients place in you" [CAN]. Recounting an incident in her work when she confronted a patient who was surreptitiously recording a consultation without asking for her permission, she asked: "In the private sector, would you dare to go head-to-head with a patient who is audiorecording you? [...] You might really just let them audiorecord you. Everything will be said in a bureaucratic manner. You wouldn't have a very pure doctor-patient relationship" [CAN].

Solitary Practice

In private practice in Hong Kong, doctors are often individually in charge of patients, with little scope for collaborating with other doctors in the management of patients. Several doctors thought of this as a serious disadvantage. One doctor said: "There are things that we can't do in the private sector, because in the private sector it's a 'one-man band'" [CAN]. Another doctor also used the English phrase "one-man band" to describe work in the private sector, saying that there,

> The challenge is that you are a "one-man band." That is, your patient is yours, and you follow up on them until they don't want you, or you don't want them. It's very clingy, basically. If anything comes up with the patient, they may immediately call you. I know my own personality. I care a lot, so I'm afraid that I would [...] stay at the hospital all the time and not be able to come home. Also, this would be relatively boring, because you're kind of on your own. Although the entire private hospital has many doctors, many in fact work very independently, without much teamwork. I don't like this very much. [...] In public hospitals, you see a case as a team, and you work on something as a team, so the atmosphere is different. [CAN]

A third doctor who used the same phrase "one-man band" explained that "[i]n our [specialist unit], we work 'more' as a 'team,'" whereas "you wouldn't have several private doctors to 'manage' one patient. So outside, it's definitely a 'one-man band'" [CAN].

2.3.1.3 Work Benefits

This category is distinguished from the previous category of "ideals and meanings in work" by its greater focus on relatively more objective attributes of public hospital work, rather than an emphasis on the subjective interpretation of aspects of public hospital work. However, this is, as with all categories and themes in this chapter, a matter of degree rather than of absolute distinction, since whether a particular aspect of work is considered a benefit or not must still be based on a person's individual understanding.

Income and Employment Security

Unlike in the private sector where doctors may need to worry about setting up and maintaining their business, being a doctor in public hospitals is a highly stable job and comes with a steady, predictable income. A number of doctors mentioned this as an appealing feature. One doctor said: "I'm inclined towards a job with a little bit more stability" [CAN]. He also thought: "I don't have financial or family reasons to immediately rush out there into the 'private' sector. So why don't I stay here first? And ultimately, this is a 'stable' job" [CAN]. Another doctor said:

> I'm not the kind of person who likes "change." I prefer more stability. First, I've already become used to the environment in this job. Out there, if I had to establish my own career, [...] it would be like "build[ing]" a "business." This would be to "take [a] risk," and there's a chance of losing, or you need to be defensive at the beginning. You may not earn as much as you imagined. So I'm a little bit hesitant about this. [CAN]

A third doctor said: "My 'personal reason' is because ultimately there's 'stability' in government [work]. [...] It's a 'comfort zone'—not very 'comfort[able],' but still a 'comfort zone'" [CAN]. A fourth doctor made very similar points: "After working here for so long, it's my 'comfort zone.' I'm not very 'sure' what 'uncertaint[ies]' there might be if I go out [into the private sector] now. [...] So I haven't gathered the courage to take this step" [CAN].

Although public hospital doctors' salaries may not be as high as those of some of their private sector colleagues, several doctors commented that their salaries were still reasonably generous. One doctor said:

> "HA" salaries are not bad. To be honest, compared with those in many other "profession[s]," they can be considered very high. The "salary" is very "stable," and the "prospect" is "foreseeable": you can see what it will be like for you in the next 10 years. And, for instance, you have over 20 days of "annual leave," like civil servants. This is already quite a lot. When you are on leave from the "HA," it's real leave. You can drop everything and won't need to "worry about" your "clinic" having to pay rent or that type of thing. So for me, for now, there's nothing that can move me. I think my life is very "balanced" and "stable." So I will stay with the "HA." [CAN]

Another doctor said: "In Hong Kong, the HA system's pay is probably one of the highest in the world. So if you have very realistic or monetary concerns, I think staying in the public system is okay." A third doctor commented: "In the end those who stay with the Hospital Authority may be those who hope to live comfortably, who by nature want a life where you clock in and out of work, or those who love to do hospital administration work" [CAN].

Case Complexity and Variation

This theme is closest to the previous theme of "patients from all walks of life." However, the quotations here focus more on the variety and complexity of medical conditions that patients in the public system have, and how treating such conditions benefited doctors' case exposure, skill progression, experience, and sense of professional satisfaction, and less on how treating underprivileged patients from all social backgrounds gave doctors a sense of personal fulfilment.

One doctor said that in his particular subspecialty, "Outside [in the private sector], many things do not 'support' 'major surger[ies]' or 'complicated surger[ies].' You can't do it. There's no 'ICU' support. [...] Of course there are many types of simple procedures, [...] but there is a very large 'spectrum' of very rare procedures'" [CAN].

A second doctor said: "The most serious cases 'end up' in the public system. [...] I myself am inclined towards wanting to see and handle more complex cases" [CAN]. A third doctor said: "To be honest, if you go out into the private sector, you'll handle some low-risk things. I myself am a bit more 'adventurous,' and I want to do those relatively higher risk surgeries, 'which' is 'part' of the 'job satisfaction' that the private sector cannot give me" [CAN]. A fourth doctor said: "The 'case[s]' that are the most difficult to handle or the most complex usually go to university hospitals or 'tertiary referral centre[s].' [...] I 'specialize' in relatively more complex [specialist procedure], and these are usually 'high risk.' Those are usually performed at university hospitals" [CAN]. A fifth doctor said: "In the public system, apart from helping others, it's also 'for' myself, because ultimately 90% of 'patient[s]' are in the public system. In particular, I'm at [a specific hospital], and before we would get many patients referred to us [with] some very strange diseases, some very 'complex'." [CAN].

The challenge posed by very acute and urgent cases, which tend not to be accepted by private hospitals, gave doctors some of their most memorable professional experiences, and kept them in the public system despite some of the other benefits of the private sector. One doctor said:

> Handling very urgent "case[s]," or having to handle a very "ill patient" suddenly [...] [and] being able to "handle" it in the end, working successfully on a "case" with the whole "team"—I do feel "satisfaction." When I can help patients, I will feel this is "why my life is a life." [...] In fact, I've considered going to the "private" sector, but I think that I won't be able to have as much "job satisfaction" there. "To be honest," I would perhaps have to "give up" these things, but I would have [...] "more flexibility and time." [CAN]

She elaborated:

> Throughout my career perhaps there were two to three times when I felt I really saved a patient. For instance, once [...] there was a patient with a [particular disease] in the "ICU." [...] At that moment I needed to quickly make a "diagnos[is]," ask the "trainee" to get medication to [treat a specific problem], perform CPR on the "patient," and "resuscitate" the patient after cardiac "arrest." It wasn't just me but the whole "ICU" "team['s] teamwork." [...] We successfully resuscitated her, and she woke up. In such "instance[s]" I think, "I really saved someone." There aren't many of such cases, but I think that if I wasn't at a "public hospital," I wouldn't be able to handle such "case[s]." [CAN]

Increasing Autonomy and Ownership with Seniority

As doctors completed their training, they took more individual charge over patients under their care, rather than being only responsible for small parts of patient care during their training. This led to a greater sense of autonomy and job satisfaction for some doctors. One doctor said:

> I think my "job satisfaction" was slowly "buil[t]" up "over" six years of "training." As a fellow I've worked for almost five years. When I can "handle" my own "case[s]," my "job satisfaction" is even higher. Before, I didn't really think about the meaning of being a doctor, because I was "training" and sitting exams continuously. [...] Sometimes, with some small cases, I felt like I was really "manag[ing]" a "case" and thinking of a "patient" as my patient.

> But obviously, after having become a fellow, with "completely independent practice" in these past five years, there have been more of such "case[s]" [CAN].

Another doctor said that as his seniority increased, "I get to deal with other things, which are perhaps a bit more fulfilling in terms of trying to see a patient get better." A third doctor said: "I think after working around 11 or 12 years, I started to become 'independent.' Starting from that time, gradually as you work on difficult 'case[s],' or work on very urgent 'case[s],' you get a sense of achievement" [CAN].

Having junior doctors assist them with the more basic tasks also meant that doctors had more time to forge deeper connections with patients. One doctor said that as a "junior," doing ward rounds,

> In one day, you would see 30 cases in one go. [...] So you wouldn't have time to slowly chat with the "patient" or to "build up" the "relationship." Now, I still need to do ward rounds, but a "junior" will already have done the ward round, so when I go there I will in fact already have an understanding of what has happened to them so far. So I can have more direct communication with them. I like what I do now more than what I used to. I think the communication has improved. [CAN]

He elaborated:

> This is a problem with the whole public system. The more "junior" [doctors] are extremely busy, but the more "senior" [doctors] are not as busy. [...] Now that I have a little bit more time to "build" a "rapport" with patients, I think I'm quite satisfied with current conditions. But this really only comes to pass when you have enough staff. It just so happens that recently, my team has somewhat more staff, so I can do this. Compared with when I was a "junior," my team has double the number of people now, so it's more comfortable. [...] When you have more time, you can spend more time on each patient. [CAN].

Further Training and Enhanced Learning

Related to the theme of "case complexity and variation" is the view that there were many more prospects for further learning in the public system. This was appealing to doctors who felt, like one doctor did, that "What I feel I need to do the most is 'lifelong learning'" [CAN]. This doctor thought:

> "Throughout" these 10 years, the "direction" of the "medical field," whether it's in terms of "research" or "practice," has undergone big changes. So "lifelong learning" is very important. For instance, before, the emphasis was very much on the "clinical" side, on treating patients in a hands-on way. But now, with "technolog[ical]" advances, for instance in "genetics," "genomics," or "big data study," ways to "apply techniques" to the treatment of patients is very different from 10 years ago. The only thing that hasn't changed is that patients need "comfort." [CAN]

Another doctor agreed that further training was essential. She explained:

> These few years we've been to India quite a few times, because India's development [in a type of specialist surgery] is very "advanced." [...] We went there to learn some new types of surgery, and then we took these back to Hong Kong, and successfully helped some patients in Hong Kong [to recover]. I think these are the meanings I can find in my work. [CAN]

A third doctor said:

> For me [encountering rare and complex cases in the public system] is a type of... [...] learning, for the further improvement of my "skills." [This is] because for a "surgeon," studying means "knowledge," but a large part [of being a surgeon] is about experience, about the hands, about working in the "OT." Only by doing, by actual doing, can you learn those "skills" and "tricks." These are areas that public hospitals will continuously "train" someone in, and areas where I will continuously "modify" myself and do learning in. [CAN]

The doctor who was quoted under the theme of "commercial interests" under the category of "problems in the private sector" on an instance when she was secretly audiorecorded during a consultation discussed the less formal ways of learning that the public system provided her:

> If I wasn't in this industry, then when I face a patient who is audiorecording me, I might not have the opportunity to reflect on how to handle things when encountering this situation. [...] I don't know how to "verbalize" or "articulate" what type of benefit this is, but I think it's quite important. It can perhaps lead to my "mentality" becoming even more mature, me being able to "handle" even more "crises," and having more "perspective[s]" in my thinking. And my own value system, centered on pursuing "kindness," is now clearer. You can even say [it is] to "promote kindness." [...] Being a doctor brings me many benefits for my personal growth, so perhaps my gain in this area is an invisible "pull factor," "pull[ing]" at me to stay here. [CAN]

Working for a large organization like the Hospital Authority also provides more protection from risk, which in turn leads to more learning opportunities, as another doctor commented:

> The Hospital Authority allows us to develop [in a variety of ways]. That is, if there are new techniques, then in private hospitals, you might be concerned about what would happen if anything happened to patients. But public hospitals are government organizations, so as long as you get past some administrative aspects, that is they "approve" you trying out this thing, the hospital will help you handle some problems that might appear. So you can try new things with more courage. [CAN]

This doctor was therefore able to introduce a new specialist procedure in Hong Kong:

> One year before I took my exams in my specialty, I brought a non-invasive [specialist surgical procedure] to Hong Kong. I was the first one to perform this surgery in Hong Kong that year, [...] so I brought this skill here. Now it's so common that everyone thinks this is the norm. [...] My sense of achievement from this was quite big. In terms of my career, this was a very "technical" advancement. [CAN]

She pointed out that after completing specialist training, there are also opportunities to "develop our own subspecialty," which she availed herself of by going overseas to learn a particular type of specialist surgery. Another doctor mentioned being able to shape his subspecialty to maximize her impact: "I'm glad that there's an opportunity for my team, to allow me to develop the subspecialty [...] into something that I feel that I can contribute to."

One doctor, like the doctor quoted in the last paragraph, spoke of the importance of overseas training to her:

> I went overseas on and off for three to four months. It was like a "break," giving me some time off from the things in Hong Kong. It was purely to go overseas to see what other people did.. [...] Since that "overseas training," my mentality has changed. It's because after you leave for a while, you can see things more clearly. [CAN]

She also found the availability of the specialist equipment in the public system appealing, describing a specialist hospital she first visited and later started work at as "like a new place that allowed me to 'explore' more different 'option[s].' For instance, there was some new 'equipment' I could use, new 'service[s]' that I could bring in to this hospital [...]. So I thought, why not continue to give it a few more years here?" [CAN].

Four doctors were forthright about the need that doctors had to gain experience as one of the main reasons for why some doctors chose to remain in the public system for the time being. One said: "I think most doctors stay in the public system either because they want to serve the patients or they're still kind of developing their skills [...]. They want to be very independent before they go to the private sector" [CAN]. Another doctor also said: "In [my specialty], I think I need a little bit more 'experience,' so I think the main reason why I'm staying is because of 'experience'" [CAN]. A third doctor repeated this view, saying that doctors in her specialty "need a little bit more time to 'build up experience'" [CAN], although apart from this more pragmatic concern, she also felt a deep sense of achievement from this process: "the real 'satisfaction' is from my 'surgical skills' [...] continuously improving" [CAN]. A fourth doctor pointed out that the reason why doctors worked for public hospitals was "not because one wants to selflessly sacrifice oneself. This would not be the true story. The true story is that we must. If we want to become a specialist doctor, or we need more experience, we would definitely choose to work at a public hospital" [CAN].

Research Work

Closely related to the previous theme was doctors' wish to conduct research alongside their clinical duties, often in order to make a greater impact on society and for the advancement of medical science. This is frequently part of doctors' work at public hospitals. One doctor said: "I like the 'research' here, the teaching. So that's why again I say that I don't necessarily need to go out to make money" [CAN]. Another doctor said that although "there were people who were trying to coax me into the private sector, I 'turn[ed]' it 'down.' The main reason was because actually, our 'team' has a very 'strong' 'academic basis.' There was such 'exposure' right upon joining the 'team'" [CAN]. He thought that ultimately, "'university hospitals' have their 'edge.' Although it's definitely busier from the very beginning, [...] the way I look at it is that being 'nurture[d]' in the 'best environment' always has its appeal" [CAN]. A third doctor said: "I want to make 'advance[s]' in this profession, to do more 'research.' This is in fact very difficult in the private sector. In the public sector, especially in university hospitals, it's easier. I know that some private doctors do research, but the 'limitation' is very big" [CAN]. The space for this arose after he passed his specialist exams:

> My direction has not really changed. I still want to learn how to help people. At this moment, I've passed my exams, so I'm thinking about how to do a little bit more, to do new things in my own profession, to give my peers more insight, or to come to new "findings" to lead this profession to the next step, so it's a bit different. Before I was learning to "follow" the "system," and now I'm learning how to "build" something new on top of this "system," or change current 'guideline[s]' [...]. Of course not everyone thinks like this. I know some people who purely want to "practice medicine" to help people, and that's it. I'm more inclined towards doing a bit more research [...]. Before, I would rely on my pair of hands, and now, apart from my pair of hands, I want to do more "evidence-base[d]" things to help even more people "make a decision." [CAN]

A fourth doctor emphasized how research could help spread knowledge beyond Hong Kong. She said:

> The "case[s]" we see are too "complicated" and "rare," particularly when we're talking about performing [a specific type of] "surgery," which in the whole of Hong Kong only we do, [and which] many South-East Asian countries don't do. But when you "share" your "experience," [...] even when it's just a plain "case report," [...] we hope that we can help others see that there are such "case[s]" that can be looked at in these ways. [...] So this is something else that makes me feel that by staying at public hospitals, at teaching hospitals, I have more opportunities to do such things, giving me another type of fulfilment. [CAN]

A fifth doctor discussed the importance of developing research knowledge tailored to the Hong Kong context. He said:

> Perhaps there is a disease which, in the context of Hong Kong, you don't know the "outcome" of [...]. You can reference overseas [research], [...] but "those are not Hong Kong people, those are not Chinese" [people]. That means that if you can gain some experience in Hong Kong, and then apply this to your everyday "clinical practice," this is quite useful.

In addition, he pointed out that "because our supervisors are very renowned in the field [...] they can lead us who are in the 'mid[dle] levels' [...] to go out and get in contact with doctors from different places. These things I believe would be difficult in private practice" [CAN].

Empowering Teamwork

As discussed under the theme "solitary private practice," whereas in private practice, doctors tend to take charge of the care of individual patients and earn income directly from this, in public hospitals, doctors need to work together to serve the majority of the population. Many doctors discussed this as a significant advantage. One doctor said:

> In public hospitals there's the advantage that there are so many "team[s]," so we can work together on many things. For instance, I have patients whom I treat with rheumatologists, and patients whom I treat with neurologists, or with endocrinology—"anytime I can find help within the hospital." [...] We have different 'subspecialt[ies],' and we can develop our own, so that within each "field" we can gain even greater familiarity with diseases or

"treatment[s]," and can be the most "up to date." [...] When I encounter some cases [of specific diseases], I can feel secure about "refer[ring]" these to my colleagues to "manage" these, or [in the knowledge that] they can give a very good "opinion" on how to "treat" such patients. [CAN]

Another doctor said that "if you compare 'teamwork' with setting up your own practice, where you shoulder everything, then you can see the benefits of 'teamwork.' And you can learn a lot from everyone around you, for instance how your 'senior' handles a case, or you can also observe how others handle it." [CAN]. That was why she thought: "If I can handle the 'work-health balance' here, I'm eager to continue my work as a doctor in the form of 'teamwork,' continuing to learn and improve" [CAN].

Teamwork also offered doctors collegial and mental support when handling challenging cases or when going through a rough patch. One doctor said: "The challenges of your public hospital work are not so great that you feel like they're not manageable. [...] And I think my team is very supportive. So you always feel like you can fall back on someone else's help if you encounter any difficulties." Another doctor said:

I like working together with different "parties." It's fun. And often when we exchange "idea[s]," you discover new ways of thinking. [...] I love "teamwork." I think I like coming back to the ward, and the atmosphere is such that everyone is very happy, and is "work[ing]" together like a family. I've worked with some of the assistants in the ward for over 10 years. Very often we know how to have good coordination together. I like that "dynamic" and that atmosphere. [CAN]

Two other doctors recounted how teamwork benefited specific cases they handled, making a lasting impact on the way they thought about their work. One doctor said:

My team is very good—the team spirit is very good. The vast majority of doctors care about patients. Whether they are [...] "academic[s]" or "HA" colleagues, they put patients in first place. No matter how busy they are [...], the moment they receive a "call" [...] about a surgery to be done, everyone immediately drops what they're doing to do this. [CAN]

This doctor once made a decision to treat an urgent and highly unpredictable case suddenly outside of office hours, and was fully supported by his colleagues:

When you need to "assemble" so many people in "non-office hour[s]" to help a patient with a very high mortality rate, it is very difficult. But "somehow" every single person, as soon as I called them, didn't say no. They said, "Okay. Give me 45 minutes. I'll come back to do this." [...] In the end I "assemble[d]" a "team" to come back and do this, with me as "chief operator" [...]. We did it very quickly, and after we were finished the patient [who had been in a coma] woke up "on the spot," and we took out her tube. [...] I was very "grateful" because so many people believed in my "decision" [to try and save the patient], and it wasn't just me, but the whole "team" who wanted the patient to recover and who therefore came back much earlier. Amongst them, many have children, or they have to come back at 7 am the next morning, so if they come back at 3 or 4 am, and they do the surgery till 6, then from 6 to 7 they can perhaps rest for one hour until they have to go back to work. So many people very "willingly" made different sacrifices to help the patient. I found this very touching. [CAN]

Another doctor recounted saving a patient's life even after "the whole world has said, 'that's it, there's no saving [the patient]'":

> You get people's "support," and the support of other "team[s]," and wow, you discover that it's really "amazing," that in fact life can be less easily lost, that we can do something to help someone that everyone has given up on to "survive." So I think it is very meaningful to be here. [CAN]

She elaborated on the benefits of team support:

> It's really precious to have the support of a "team." When you want to go crazy [and do something unusual]—I call it going crazy—[…] but the whole "team" actually 'support[s]' you in going crazy, and then there are other specialties, and other "professor[s]" who do something with you together, it's a very precious opportunity. I think these [opportunities] don't exist outside of big hospitals. [CAN]

Instead, in private hospitals,

> the cases you see are all "low-risk case[s]." […] It may seem like I'm describing them as very bad, referring all the "high-risk case[s]" to us. But just think about it: because we deal with many "rare" cases or cases with "complication[s]," we can't in fact handle them as individuals, but need to handle them as a "team." […] Only public hospitals have such complete facilities. So of course there are some bad "private" doctors who "refer" everything to us, but even some doctors who really care, that is you know that they treat "patient[s]" really well, and make really accurate "diagnos[es]" and so on, still face "limitation[s]" and can't do it. Then what will happen to those "patient[s]"? […] Therefore, I think this will make me feel even more that only if I "stay" can I do these things" [CAN].

"How to work as a team, how to maintain our 'team spirit': these things are very important, because as you work longer and longer, you discover many things are not just your own. […] You discover it's only when we 'work as a team' that we can do something well" [CAN]. This creates higher level meaning, one that she was not sure how to fully articulate: "when you see the team spirit, working together to do something well, no matter what the outcome—although the outcome in most cases is good—you think even more strongly that the meaning is not that simple. I don't know how to express this—my abilities of expression are not that good" [CAN].

Finally, such teamwork also furthers learning, and can therefore be seen as a continuation of the previous theme of "further training and enhanced learning." One doctor said: "Within a team there are 'junior' and 'senior' doctors, and even within the same 'subspecialty,' you can have different people to help you. So it's very suitable for 'training'" [CAN].

Treatment Detached From Commercialism

Whereas the previous theme of "commercial interests" under the category of "problems in the private system" focused on doctors describing what might happen if they practised privately, this theme lays out the quotations where the emphasis was on the benefits of the non-commercialism of treatment in public hospitals, even though interviewees might still refer briefly to what happens in the private sector. One doctor said:

> I'm able to say these cool words all the time: "This is a public hospital. I only treat and manage this disease. Although we have limited resources, we will use the best and the most 'proper' ways to treat you. Do not talk to me about money—this is irrelevant." This is something very nourishing, very real. Hong Kong is in a very fortunate position: in Hong Kong public hospitals, unless there is something that is definitely not possible in terms of resources, some very "extreme" and very advanced technology, or something that you need to take away such as coronary stents, which you must pay for yourself, then in fact many things are "up to" international "standard[s]." That is, they won't use inferior things just because you don't need to pay, or it won't be much inferior. So the standard is quite good, and you don't need to pay. So you don't have financial considerations, which for the sake of treating diseases and for learning is very good, because when you have the additional layer of financial considerations, there's a big difference. [CAN]

A second doctor also said:

> If you are my "patient," when I discuss the condition of your [specific organ] with you, I don't need to think about anything to do with money. I only need to talk to you about what the benefits and drawbacks of something are to you, and options "ABC," and what is good about "A" or "B" or "C." I don't need to tell you how much "A" or "B" or "C" costs, because to me, this makes no difference. The money does not go directly into my pocket. The "Hospital Authority" pays me a salary. So no matter what I do, I will have that money, and I won't get more or less. [CAN]

He compared the treatment options in the private sector with those in the public sector for his specialty:

> Because of the cost of the medication, many chronically ill patients would find it very tough to receive treatment in the private sector. [...] But in public hospitals, this is not a very big "concern," because the medicine is funded by the government. We have many medicines to choose from, and patients would not need to have a big "financial burden." [CAN]

A third doctor similarly said: "I'm not sure how much you can give back to society once you're in private practice. It's more like a business [there]. In the public sector, I think that the best part of it is that I don't have to think about cost. I can just give whatever I think is appropriate for the patients."

One doctor spoke not only of it being unnecessary to lay out financial considerations to patients, but also of being able to be much more truthful to the patient when compared with doctors in private practice, who might need to keep silent on some matters out of commercial interests:

> If there's something that shouldn't be done like this, of course you will tell the patient. You can be tactful [...] or direct. In any case, I need to make them understand based on the principle behind treating the disease, if you walk the path in this way, it will be smoother—even if I need to be tactful, I must still tell them. [CAN]

She "quite 'enjoy[ed]'" such an "pure doctor-patient relationship":

> For instance, when I tell the patient that they need to do this or that, [...] or I have to do overtime because of them, I'm not doing this to earn more money off of them. I'm doing it for your illness. I don't want to delay your treatment. Or I want you to be less anxious, so I will say some comforting words. These things aren't motivated by financial considerations. So when they thank me, maybe I think that I do absolutely deserve this. [...] This is because I understand that my intention is really to help them, and not to ingratiate myself with them" [CAN].

Like the doctor quoted in the first paragraph, she pointed out that "we receive a 'fixed amount' of 'income.' I won't, like in the private system, be nicer to you because I want to earn more money off you" [CAN].

2.3.2 *Standards of Medical Work Set by Doctors*

In the interviews, many doctors mentioned work standards they either started their career with or developed throughout their career, and which they held themselves to. These were benchmarks or criteria that they set for themselves in their work because they believed that not abiding by these would affect the quality of their work.

In their affiliation with the words "ideals" and "meanings," these "standards" are closely linked to some of the themes under the previous category of "ideals and meanings in work." However, the personal ideals discussed in that category represented broader, more abstract aspirational goals that doctors wanted their work to embody, which served as a guiding vision or inspiration to them. The personal meanings similarly referred more directly to the significance or values that doctors attached to their work experiences, and from which they derived fulfilment and a sense of purpose. In contrast, the standards described in this group outline how doctors felt they should act in their work roles in order to be good doctors. These standards tended to be more concrete and specific guidelines that were part of the practical, everyday context of doctors' work.

One additional crucial distinction is that the themes under "ideals and meanings in work" are distinguished from the themes grouped here because quotations under the former tended to explicitly discuss "doctor's reasons for wanting to stay on in public hospitals," which is the overarching group heading for them. Conversely, the "standards" below were benchmarks doctors set for their work with relatively little reference to these as reasons for wanting to remain in the public sector.

2.3.2.1 Bringing Patients Comfort

Two doctors pointed out that helping patients should not only take the form of providing medical treatment, but should also include bringing comfort to patients. One doctor said:

> "Bring[ing] comfort to" patients and their family: this hasn't changed in these past 10 years. We need to treat patients in a sincere and "honest" way. These "qualities" will never change. "Technology" has "advance[d]," and "attitude[s]" to "treatment options" have been constantly changing. But I think some very "core human values" will probably not change within my lifetime. [CAN]

Another doctor said:

> There's a quote which I think has been misassigned to Hippocrates, the father of medicine: [...] in our profession, we can cure sometimes, we can treat every now and then, but we

> should reassure or provide comfort in other situations always. And so that's really stuck with me, that we should try and at least do the very minimum of what doctors were supposed to do. And so that's something that I tell my residents to constantly tell themselves.

2.3.2.2 Fulfilling the Weight of Responsibility

This theme is closely related to the themes of "fulfilment from helping patients" and "duty to patients and society," but, as mentioned, as an explanation for doctors' work in general rather than as a specific reason to stay in the public sector. One doctor said:

> I've deeply felt and witnessed how big a doctor's power is. You can really dictate a patient's life or death. [...] Before, when I was [in a particular specialty], very often the patient's [specific organ] has already got very serious problems. Sometimes [...] family members will ask for a chance. Looking at it objectively, if you do surgery, you cannot help them, and they might be put in a vegetative state. Have we really helped you if you are put in a vegetative state? In fact there are many such "ethical issue[s]" to handle. But the point these issues bring out is that doctors have great power, that is our ability is great [...], and the greater your ability, the greater of course your "responsibility." [CAN]

Another doctor said:

> In this line of work, your responsibility towards patients is big. [...] You have to be meticulous about patients' situations. You have to be more careful when doing everything, to prevent yourself from making mistakes or from harming patients. This hasn't changed throughout these years, and after so many years, you'll become more careful, or think this is even more important. [CAN]

A third doctor felt that "once they are under my care, I'm 100% responsible from the first day of their hospital journey to when they get discharged." A fourth doctor spoke of fulfilling her responsibility to patients as providing both her and her patients with mental calm: "I think now I pursue patients' 'peace of mind' and my own 'peace of mind.' For instance, if I fulfil my responsibilities properly, I will feel at ease about having done things right" [CAN].

2.3.2.3 Compassionate, Effective Communication in Care

Many doctors emphasized the importance of good communication strategies with patients in order to establish an effective relationship with them. Although constraints on time mean that it can be difficult for doctors to communicate well and in a compassionate way, two doctors pointed out that just shifting one's viewpoint or approach slightly might already be sufficient in enacting the necessary improvements. One doctor said that it did not take much extra effort or time in communication to show care, but that it made a big difference:

> Actually, it's not difficult [to understand patients better]—it just depends on whether you want to or not. In fact, you just need to, when they come back for a follow-up consultation, ask them a couple more questions, [such as] "What do you want to do? What is your biggest

> expectation"? You really just need to ask a couple more questions, and often, the "patient" is very "willing" to let you know why they are so "hesita[nt]" about having surgery done, or why they want to do a surgery. [CAN]

A second doctor suggested being more aware of how each patient is a human being with their own life history. After recounting how he chatted with a lonely and seriously ill patient, he said:

> I think the biggest "impression" from this event is that sometimes when things are… not really "out of" our "comfort zone," "but out of" our usual conversational approaches, if you just say a bit more, or can "just be more curious" about the "patient," about what they themselves are thinking, or "just" as small talk… At first when I started to chat with him it wasn't for anything specific, but just because I was doing these procedures, and didn't want him them to be bored and staring at what I was doing, and make me even more "stressed." We started talking and […] it was very run-of-the mill the first few times. But subsequently you would hear about how his background was in fact very wretched. […] Very often it's the environment that influences [your situation in life]. […] Sometimes we may only see some "label[s]" that say they're an "IV drug user" and so on. We may "label" a "patient" as a miscreant. In fact, I think "at the end of the day" people are by nature benevolent, but it's just that their "circumstances" or their willpower weakened. So "even if" this is the case, I think "there's always a story behind" every person, and although understanding more may not be necessary "from a clinical point of view," "at least" you can have better "rapport" with the "patient." […] "Every patient" has a "back story behind" them. For some, their "circumstances" are unfortunate and truly awful, but "in general," I think that […] them having such ailments is in fact very often "out of" their "control." [CAN]

Other doctors also highlighted communication as able to change the entire dynamics of the doctor-patient rapport even when the objective clinical outcome was not changed. One doctor said: "Very often it depends on how you communicate with them, 'instead of' what you did" [CAN]. Another doctor said: "Apart from the disease, how to communicate with patients [is also important], because very often it's not just that I say you have this disease, so you take this medication and get treated. Patients have their 'concern[s]' and their way of thinking" [CAN]. How to meet patients' need for good communication while still being able to manage one's workload becomes a great challenge:

> Our "workload" is very big. For instance, in one shift of three hours, we need to see 20 to 30 patients. So it's five minutes per patient. Perhaps some cases are more complex, and you need to spend more time to discuss things with them. […] Some cases are simple, but the case being simple does not mean that the person is simple. So we need to learn how to use a very short amount of time to communicate with patients, and have the patient understand what we are saying, and that we're not just pushing them out. This is a struggle. [CAN]

Another doctor talked about needing to forcefully carve out more time to communicate with patients with more complex conditions and less time on others. She said:

> Normally, if they don't have anything serious, "patient[s]" will come and go very quickly, that is they really get up almost as soon as they sit down. But for some patients, you know that they really have special needs, and you really need to talk to them for very long. […] You know there are 20 or so "patient[s]" behind them, but you still need to stop everything to handle some relatively special "patient[s]." This isn't because we get along better in conversation,

> but because their illness requires me to stop and talk to them, because sometimes they really have more "complicated" [illnesses]. [CAN]

She could not spare more time for more straightforward cases, even as her own view was that "within the 'HA,' you just need to be willing to spend the time and effort to talk to [patients], and the 'difference' will already be very big" [CAN], and even as she believed in the role of communication in personalizing treatment:

> "sometimes when discussing with the 'patient' how to 'manage' them, you will think you know a lot, and that you know what to do, but [...] your treatment in fact isn't like the pure 'evidence-based treatment' that 'school' teaches you. Instead you really need to discuss with the patient what they want, to 'personalize' the whole 'management'" [CAN].

A third doctor identified a shift towards emphasizing good communication with patients throughout the past few decades, so that consultations take much more time than they used to:

> Doctors from 30 years ago were very "authoritative." When doctors told you that you should do this or that, you had to follow the instructions. But now, you have to be very clear in what you say. For instance, for performing a simple surgery, you have to talk about the "indications," and whether there is an "alternative": [...] what's the benefit of having the surgery done versus not having it done, or what the disadvantages are, or what ways there are to do the surgery. You have to be very clear in order to have what we call "informed consent." So in this regard, you will spend a lot of time. But this is because the system used to be different, with very few people, so doctors did something very quickly after talking about it, and could do the next thing. Whereas now the emphasis is on "communication" and "patient understanding." This is a big change. [CAN]

A fourth doctor similarly identified an attenuation of the authoritarianism that undergirded medical consultations and treatment in the past. He said:

> You will see patient culture having changed. The impression "patient[s]" had of doctors 10 years ago was, "I must listen to what you say, and what you say I must follow, and then things will be "okay." Even when the "result" or "outcome" is bad, it's because of me. But with more information becoming accessible, and the "culture" changing, we often say we need to "involve" "patient[s]" in the "management plan." So it's no longer me telling you this, this, this, but everyone discussing. I have an "opinion" to give you, a "choice" to give you, and you choose the "choice" that suits you the most. We face things together, and we battle the disease together. Or we go do "rehabilitation" to "achieve" a "result" that everyone considers the best result. [This is] because if it's always me saying things, and they have no say, the "result" is never going to be good. In contrast, when you "involve" them, discuss with them as equals, communicatively "involve" them, choose a "management" [path] together, and consider things while standing in their shoes, then in fact, the "outcome" is always one that makes everyone happy. [CAN]

This was the case even when "everyone knew that [the disease] would not have a good 'outcome,' that there would be 'limitation[s]'" [CAN]: he discovered, after working for three to four years, that as long as "I had this 'mindset' when I sat down to talk to a 'patient,' and 'involve[d]' a 'patient' in the 'patient management plan,' very often the 'patient' would be very 'satisfied' with the situation" [CAN]. Because of the overwhelming difference that good communication could make, he commented:

> The most important thing is to look at them when talking to them, to think from their perspective. You should not type on the computer while talking to them, because they will think that you and they are inhabiting different spaces. So I place a lot of importance on sitting down and looking at them, and then asking: "How have you been? [...] What can I help you with?" [...] In fact it's very simple, but there are time limitations. [CAN]

Some doctors also spoke of the difference their communication made to patients' emotional wellbeing. One doctor said: "'You don't need to worry'—this sentence can 'reassur[e]' patients a lot" [CAN]. Another doctor discussed his experience undergoing surgery as a patient himself. The doctor's surgeon "was there as a 'reassuring figure.' [...] When she spoke with you she was a very good 'figure,' telling you 'Don't worry, I can help.' So in my 'practice,' I also want to give the same feeling to patients" [CAN]. A third doctor discussed what approach to take on when talking to the family of patients: "At that 'moment' [of their children being ill] 'parents' are already very upset. If you still say something very provocative, you may cause them to lose 'trust'" [CAN]. A fourth doctor said she was acutely aware of how "every sentence that we doctors say really affects 'patient[s'] emotions" [CAN]. She discussed the complex tensions that she had to navigate when breaking bad news to patients:

> I have an agenda, because I'm thinking about how when I "convey" this "bad news," I don't want them to be too hopeless. [...] After over 10 years' experience, many trials and tribulations have led to one refined sentence, and I know that if I say it in this way, they will be less upset. [...] I want to "b[e] kind to them," but if I don't tell this "bad news," they will miss a... because for some diseases [...], you need to "make" a "decision" a bit earlier very often. [...] So if I'm not clear enough in what I say, they won't grasp the seriousness. If they come all the way to see me today, but aren't able to "make" a "decision," then time will pass, and their physical condition will worsen. So I may be even more impatient than them, that is, I want them to come to a decision quickly. I need to very skilfully lead them to understand the essence of very complex medical decisions and their benefits and drawbacks. [...] I need to con... not to control them, but to predict what their emotional response might be, and avoid causing them to feel hopeless as much as possible. [CAN].

Later on in the interview, she added:

> Perhaps this "kindness"... I wasn't "aware" before that I was motivated by this "kindness." So in terms especially of the language used and of communication, I put a lot of importance on how to "convey" my "message in a way that" will lead to that person being able to accept it easily, and not feel too "down." [CAN]

She did so in the hope that "they will be able to get positive energy, and understand their condition better and can be less worried" [CAN].

A third doctor discussed the importance of listening to patients' stories—even when this was not clinically relevant—in helping patients' "mental health wellbeing" [ENG], an aspect that was otherwise not directly related to her specialty. She thought that "more and more people have become aware of these issues, and so have I" [CAN], and that therefore when some of her elderly patients "start talking and can't stop, I will just let them talk for longer" [CAN]. She explained:

> I'm amongst the small number of people who have a little bit more time to listen to them talk. Other people may not be unwilling to listen to them talk, but may just not have the time to.

> [...] If I really don't have the time, I do say "I'm sorry, but I have to do some other things." But if I have the time, then why not listen? [...] Usually people talk to them for two minutes and then let them leave. They ask them about [their symptoms], and then they [the patients] leave. [...] I think for them anyone will do. As long as that person is willing to listen to them talk, they will be happy. Some inpatients are really confined and have no one to talk to. [...] Perhaps during a hospital stay of a few days, only one person talks to them, and not even for very long. So no matter what, being able to talk will make them happier. [CAN]

Two other doctors discussed the medical encounter explicitly as, using their own term, an "art" that required tailoring communication to patients' individual personalities and circumstances, and going beyond mere textbook knowledge. One doctor, who is also the second doctor quoted under this theme, said:

> Why do we say so often that "medicine" is an art? Many things aren't "black and white." Many things are a "spectrum." Because "on one side," some people are very "analytical," and before they come in, you know that they have "google[d]" everything. Perhaps they have asked three to four specialists for opinions before coming in. In fact they already have an "agenda." For those people, if they want some "facts and statistics," or "guideline[s]," then that's what you do. "That's why" we have to study a lot to "cater for" this group. But "on the other [side of the] spectrum," for some people, telling them these numbers [...] is not very important. [...] We just have to work with what we have. If their personality tends to be not so analytical, then [...] we will say: if it's like this, then "options A" and "B" would be better for you, and "C" and "D" would be worse. That is, they sometimes need a bit more "guidance," [...] and we need to be able to "switch" to doing that, to be more flexible. [CAN]

He described a case where a patient with a terminal illness that belonged to another specialty had to consult his specialty for relatively minor symptoms:

> [The symptoms] were "so low" in "priority" that when she talked about [her terminal illness], we felt obliged to help her a bit. We did our best to answer the questions she asked us. Because of this, she thought this demonstrated the most care of her problems. Whenever she came, she always had one question to ask, which was how long she still had. The [specialist doctors in charge of her terminal illness] never answered this. In fact, we have also been "train[ed]" not to answer this, because it is very difficult to specify a "deadline" for people. But one method that I myself developed was to tell her a "range," that is, we could not say "exactly" which day, "but" if you say "within days," "within weeks," and "within months," then in fact there is a rough "ballpark figure." Very often, they don't really want you to say that in September they will be gone. They want a "frame" for handling their matters after death, or maybe they have something they want to do but if they haven't reached a particular stage yet, they might think it's too "early" to do those things. To be very honest, I didn't deliberately raise these things in conversations with her, "but" she came for a follow-up consultation, and the things we had to discuss under our specialty were too unimportant. [...] So when she came in and asked these questions, we were "just obliged to" answer them. She already thought this was very good, because on the other side the answer she would get was always, "We can't say. We'll have to see [how the treatment goes]." The problem was that "this is not exactly what they want" [ENG]. I think from an observer's perspective, we could see this more clearly. [CAN].

Another doctor thought similarly that "'medicine' is in fact a 'combination of art and science.' When seeing a doctor, often you admire them for their 'communication skills.' They can really see what is causing you discomfort, rather than them teaching you to do this, this, and this" [CAN]. She recounted how offhand remarks her patient's caregiver made during a consultation led to her being able to suggest a minor but life-changing surgery for the patient: "It turns out that just some simple words, if you 'miss' them, then you will also miss out on such a small surgery. [...] One such small surgery is in fact enough to change his whole life" [CAN]. Therefore, she even thought that practising medicine was "an 'art more than [a] science'" [ENG]:

> Think about the story I just told you: just one look, and speech that indicated both the desire and hesitation to talk, leading to "communication" between you. And then because of this "communication," and your handicraft [that is, the surgery the doctor performed], leading them to [get better] again. The whole situation has "none of the science inside." You can't hear any "science" in this. [CAN]

2.3.2.4 Balancing Empathy and Its Limits

Very closely related to the above theme were doctors' discussions on the importance of empathy towards patients as a standard and foundation for not only better patient care, but also for a better understanding of the type of doctor they wanted to be, and how to be an even better one. If the starting point is the patient's perspective instead of the doctor's own, a doctor's entire perspective shifts, as one doctor explained:

> You should think about the "patient['s]" feelings. I think if you try to "shift" your feelings onto patients, you think about what feelings they have first. If the "clinic" is constantly trying to chase you away, maybe you.... In fact, the same words but said in a different tone [...], or saying a few simple sentences—I think the "impact" is very big on you. That is, your "impact" on others is very big. So I think that I shouldn't be too egocentric, and lay down my ego and try and understand. This is empathy [...], where you understand what people's feelings are. I think this is very important. [CAN]

He elaborated:

> Maybe seeing a "patient" is just a job. But when "patient[s]" see us, perhaps they have waited for a long time to be able to see us, or perhaps to them the "treatment" is a "life and death treatment," or it really "affect[s]" their whole "family planning" and their entire lives. Conversely, from my perspective, perhaps they are only one amongst the 30 "patient[s]" in my "clinic." But if you try and think from their perspective, you will discover that your importance in their lives is huge. [...] So every time I remind myself of this, that is every time I'm unhappy when doing a "procedure," or go through a very tough period, I think: "Try to think from the patient's perspective." To them, the "procedure" can be equal to their everything. This gives me a lot "motivation," "push[ing]" me to continue to do a bit better. I don't dare say that, like a saint, I do everything excellently, and that there are no "complication[s]" from any of the "surger[ies]." But I will "keep" this "incentive" when doing things. [CAN]

Another doctor also described how crucial it was for disease management to start from the patient's viewpoint:

> Each type of [a specific illness] has many different ways of treatment. Which type is the best for a "patient"? You have to sit down and talk to them, and you have to stand in their shoes, letting them know you are helping them. If you say to them, "If it's like this you don't need surgery," but from their perspective, [they think:] I'm a sportsperson, or I'm a wage earner, and I have to quickly get surgery to earn money for my family—in such cases, they will think that you don't understand them, and everyone's relationship breaks down. [CAN]

Therefore, the ultimate question for him was: "What do [patients] really need? That also means that doctors in fact are not necessarily placed very high up. They don't have to be 'professor[s]' to help people. In fact, standing at the front line, if you can think from the 'patient['s]' perspective, then the 'patient' will understand" [CAN].

A third doctor said that her own life experience had deepened her ability to empathize with patients:

> I also matured, I guess. I got married. I have my own family, so as your life experiences grow, it makes it a little bit easier for you to think in other people's shoes. I think when I was a lot younger, a lot of things were not really my concern. But now a patient sometimes says: "I have a family of my own." If I see a pediatric patient, I can imagine [him or her] as my kid. I see older patients now. My parents are older. Sometimes I can imagine it could be my parents going through that. So I think that helps with the empathy part.

Because she had "more time on my hands to try and help individual patients," she had "the luxury of being able to" empathize with patients. This was something "quite important to her," which she described as "driv[ing] my work." Although she imagined having the space to empathize with patients was "important to a lot of people as well," she pointed out that "whether you can afford to do that is another question." Her view was that "empathy for me helps rather than hinders," although "having done this job for a while, it's quite important that you separate yourself," that "you include yourself but at the same time, after having those emotions, you should be able to separate yourself from it. Otherwise you can't do your job."

Other doctors echoed these thoughts on both the importance of empathy and the need for limits to empathy to be in place in order for them to function well as doctors. One doctor described this as the various contradictory positions that doctors needed to balance themselves between:

> On the one hand you are very "attached to" your "patient[s]." On the other hand you must "detach" yourself, or else you can't continue to work. So although you are in the relationship of a patient and a doctor, there can't be too many personal emotions. Sometimes it's very difficult to "strike" a "balance." [...] But we have to maintain the right doctor-patient relationship no matter what. That is, you can't "intrude" on their personal lives. On the one hand, you have to understand them. On the other hand, you can't get too involved. So this is relatively difficult. [CAN]

Another doctor had the following advice to give to medical students as a useful rule of thumb:

> I think everyone's starting point is to help "patient[s]." Everyone says this. But I think a bit more "concrete" [advice]—and this is not just a question of "empathy"—is: if this "patient"—although you don't know her—were your "relative," then what would you do? What do you think she would "expect from" the medical system, or from the "clinical team"? Very often, if this were your relative, you would definitely not do this. [...] Of course, we also have our "limitations," because of our resources, and often there's the problem of "waiting time[s]." But in areas within our control, at least in the way we engage with people, we should communicate with them, and explain to them that the appointment is in two years and there's nothing to be done about that. So how to explain things clearly; whether they would have "alternatives"; and whether they would consider private treatment: these things "establish rapport" and communication with them. If you, with your hand on your heart, ask "If this was my relative, how would they expect [me] to conduct [my]self?" [ENG], [...]

> [and] if you can treat all patients equally, then "in general you wouldn't be too off the mark" [ENG]. [CAN]

However, he similarly suggested important limitations to empathy:

> Although you say you need "empathy," you also need to strike a "balance." […] "Empathy['s]" "definition" in English is "standing in people's shoes" [ENG]. "But" sometimes, for some things, you can't really stand entirely there. You need to be a bit "impartial," and tell them… that is, for some things they in fact want you to "list" "options in" a relatively "impartial" way, and then they make their decision. […] "At the end of the day," the decision is up the "patient and relatives" to make. No matter how engaged we are—and this is perhaps very "contradictory"—while being "empath[etic]," you need to have some "impartial[ity]" at suitable moments, that is, to do the role that they want us to take on the most. "That could be either" a completely "impartial": "option A, B, and C: you choose." "Or" maybe they cannot make a choice at all. Then you must also take a further step, and say, "Then we think 'A' would be the best. Do you agree?'" [CAN]

A third doctor also examined the boundaries of empathy in her particular line of work. She said:

> Sometimes, some very passionate colleagues want to do a lot, but they aren't aware that when you help people too much, they will develop a kind of dependency. So I think about how to help them, how to "promote" walking down their path to them. Because in some cases, they are too dependent. […] Perhaps they encounter some problems and don't know how to handle them, so they go back to that doctor. This dependency is not very healthy. I think they use doctors as life buoys. When I always grab onto the doctor for everything, then some relatively "junior" colleagues—their starting point is very good, they are passionately trying to help them, but they aren't quite aware that when they do some things, they will cause the patient to imperceptibly develop a reliance on them. But they will leave one day, because they can't always follow [patients]. And when they leave, then what? [CAN]

The limits she placed were thus there not because she did not wish to help, but to enable her to do so in the best way possible:

> As a doctor, of course you want to help people. […] [However,] thinking about this in another way, it's that we make their problems in life our responsibility. Sometimes I talk to "trainees" and tell them that it's very good that they want to help them, but their problems in life are not our responsibility as doctors to solve and handle. If not, the wrong message is imperceptibly given to patients—not one that is verbalized, but sensed by them through our attitude and feelings: that if I have problems in life, I can come back and see the doctor. And I throw those objects, those balls, at you, for you to solve. This is what I just now said would lead to a type of dependency. […] If we as doctors need to "keep" the "boundary," we need to reflect. In fact, it is impossible for us to "take" away all of the patients' problems in life. We know they have problems, and we hope that we can use our methods and see if there are any suggestions to help them. But ultimately they have to face this themselves, and handle it. I can give advice, and when you are very tired I can give you some encouragement, but "at the end of the day" the ball is in your own court. […] You can imagine if I think that their problems in life are my responsibility as a doctor, and they can't handle it, I would be very "frustrated," and think: "Why isn't it working? Did I do something not very well? Or what is it?" In reality, this isn't the case. [CAN]

One other doctor recounted a scene showing an empathic doctor in a TV series she watched and how this influenced her own work:

> Because the "prognosis" for [this disease] was very bad, after she [the actor in her role as a doctor] told the "couple" the overall "message," she went to the back stairs and cried. I thought at the time that this was how I imagined [that particular specialty] and good doctors to be like, because that doctor could experience in her heart the plight of the people she had to "interact" with. So every step she took was because she very much understood their pain. Every treatment decision that that doctor made for them, every recommendation, I think would be for "the best" for that couple. [CAN]

Therefore, although "some people ask whether being a doctor means you become numb," she found that "I myself think that I cry even more easily" [CAN]. Her ability to be emotionally attuned to herself and her patients had intensified, instead of diminished, with her years of experience:

> These 10 years, my "awareness" of my own "emotion[s]" has become much stronger. [...] I have become more and more sensitive, and my thinking more and more nuanced, with richer emotions. So I believe this is my "unintentional" gain, leading me to be more sensitive to other people's emotions. So that's why in my explanations to family or patients, I adjust my language so that they will feel that it's more comfortable to listen to—it's because of my sensitivity. [CAN]

She described a time in her own career when she felt the urge to cry over a patient's plight:

> I held back my tears, because the feeling we doctors give others is that we must "b[e] tough and strong." And I'm guiding patients through a very challenging situation. "Mostly" we should not have such "negative emotion[s]" visible on our faces. So in these past 10 years, perhaps I learned the best I could not to cry in front of patients. [CAN]

The patient, she recounted,

> knew that I had understood his thoughts. But I didn't want to "share" my most real, even "sad[der]" "emotion[s]" with him. I thought that knowing that I had understood him could already "soothe" his mind. I usually bear the even more "negative" thinking and emotions that followed on my own. I also didn't want the colleagues on my ward to know. [CAN]

Like the doctors quoted before, therefore, she placed certain limits on empathy, in her case not on feeling it, but on showing it:

> A very emotionally sensitive doctor is, I think, quite suitable for [my particular specialty]. But they must also be "mentally" quite "tough" and "strong." That is, I wouldn't feel like a failure for almost crying in the ward. I just needed to protect my professional image. [...] I'm not entirely averse to this [feeling negative emotions due to a patient's plight], because I very much accept that I am moved by patients' "suffering" to experience "negative emotions." I can tolerate this side of me. It's just that I required my professional image not to be affected, because that would affect the patient: he would question whether this doctor was reliable, and he would be even more scared." [CAN]

Her "starting point is that of 'kindness'[,] [...] to not let 'patient[s]' feel upset because of me" [CAN]. Similar to some of the previous doctors quoted, this doctor also thought that empathy enhanced her work and values: "The goal in life that is being chased: within it, do we only care about our own interest? Or do we usually think about others' interests as well? Those people are happier in their work, and more successful" [CAN].

Two doctors spoke of times when they empathized so much with patients that their own mental wellbeing was adversely affected. One doctor described a patient who was under her care for a very long time, leading to her becoming too emotionally invested: "From that case on, I thought that I really needed to learn not to become so 'attached'" [CAN]. Another doctor stressed that "empathy for patients, just really listening to them" was crucial, because "there's just so much to do that we don't listen to patients anymore, and we try to interview and cut short the conversation to get to the next... to end the consultation and move on." However, emotional engagement also at times threatened to overwhelm him. The challenge was to remain *em*pathic (of putting himself in his patient's shoes) without being overwhelmed by *sym*pathy (of being emotionally affected by his compassion for his patients):

> There is a very fine line from when I deal with [...] patients [to] overstep[ping] into sympathy. [...] But I always constantly have to tell myself that most of these patients are young—the youngest I had was six—and only have less than a year to live, so every memory counts, and I can take it quite personally in terms of what they've been going through. And it's always a process where I need to process this information, process their outcomes and inevitably, [the disease] will take their lives in less than a year. [...] It's really about trying to make sure that I have good mental health as well. Because it's tough. [CAN]

He described a time when he could no longer perform an operation because of his overwhelming sympathy for a patient who came from a socially deprived background and was terminally ill:

> I just couldn't take it anymore because this was a person that I'd been following—echoing back to the empathy-sympathy threshold, which I'd inadvertently crossed. And I said: "I can't do this operation anymore. [...] I don't want to cut into [the patient] anymore."
>
> So one of my assistants, who is as experienced as I am, said, "Don't worry. You go out. We'll do it." [...] That was the only time when I said I refused to do the surgery. I mean, I was at the table, was scrubbed in, but then I just could not [...] put knife to skin. And I essentially broke down at that point. And I said: "yeah, I can't do this." [CAN]

He described his feelings when this patient passed away: "You know, this is something where it's a personal... Now that experience... I've had many others close to this, but not quite as impactful."

The distinction between empathy and sympathy that he referred to earlier was further used by him to articulate the boundary that could be harmful to him when crossed:

> That empathy-sympathy [division]: I'm still trying to find where that line should be drawn. [...] I think the line is getting clearer and clearer to me. [...] Once it starts to affect me in a way where I'm not productive anymore and it's affecting the people that I care about as well. So where I feel: okay, I'm taking too much time out from my personal life to care for someone; where, even though I do know that there are probably not going to be that many people out there that will be able to help this person, I got to stop when it's encroaching against my personal life or the people that care for me. And so it's getting clear. I'm not saying it is absolutely clear, but then it's getting clearer and clearer to me that that's where I should draw my boundaries, because it's tough.

Based on his experience with processing these emotions, he had specific advice for trainees and students:

I do encourage residents and medical students to process this. Don't avoid it. Work through it. They'll look the other way. Look it straight in the eye. This is a young person that's going to die. This person you're going to make friends with is going to die in nine months. But this is the deal. You're becoming a doctor. That's what you need to deal with. But process it. Feel sad about it, but then quickly climb up that hole as soon as possible because you got the next patient in mind, and it could affect your mental health as well. But processing it means that you're still human. [...] I do understand there are quite a few public hospital doctors that perhaps from a... either because of work or because of a self-defence mechanism, they tend to fishbowl themselves so that they don't become too close with patients because the toll is... the price is too high. But we know that's inevitably human, so I tend to say, "I'm glad that you're crying now. I'm glad that you feel sad, because that means you're human. Experience it, and then work through it. But you have to cry quickly, then get back on your feet.

Residents actually do feel that they're always going to be, that they... they're young, right, [...] they're sharp as a whip, [...] [and] they've got their whole career ahead of them. They're gradually improving on their surgical skills. So they have that ego being built up. But then it's a very humbling subspecialty. [...] Because I always think about Susan Sontag's quote. [...] I always tell them because I know this by heart: 'everyone who is born holds dual citizenship, in the kingdom of the well and in the kingdom of the sick. Although we all prefer to use the good passport [...], sooner or later, each [...] of us is obliged, at least for a spell, to identify ourselves as citizens of that other place.' I think that's something we have to know: that we're human, and we get sick. Do you want your doctor to be just the same as you are now to treat you? Do you want your doctor to be as nonchalant, as distant, as uncaring as you are right now?

2.3.2.5 Humility

There is some overlap between this theme and the previous one on empathy, since humility may be predicated on not conceiving of the self as superior to laypersons, but on the same level. For instance, the views expressed by the last doctor quoted under the above theme who called his subspecialty "humbling" positioned empathy and humility alongside each other.

Indeed, the first two of the following three doctors quoted also mentioned being empathic to patients' needs when discussing the importance of levelling the doctor-patient hierarchy. One doctor said:

When I first graduated and started working in this field, this career was to me very mysterious, and difficult to get to know, because this is after all a very specialized field. [...] Before you have stepped foot in it, you will have a lot of fantasies about this field. In particular, from many TV programs, many things I watched, I thought this field was very "professional," with many things very "elegant," very beautiful, helping those in urgent situations and in distress. When I first started, I also had this fantasy, and thought that I had entered a new stage in life, and it was wonderful. But once you start the work, you will discover that in this field, you cannot put yourself in a very esteemed position. On the contrary, you need to think from patients' perspectives.

This is where I feel in these past 10 years or so, my mentality has changed. The younger you are, the more you think that being a doctor or being in a "medical" profession is something very esteemed, very "above," very "superior." But in fact when you really start working, you will discover that you must chat with "patient[s]" in a very down-to-earth way to understand them, and only then can you really help them. [...] So I discovered that being a doctor was not

> such a "superior" profession. In contrast, in this profession, you have to be sufficiently down-to-earth, able to understand together with "patient[s] what they are "suffer[ing]" through, and only then can you really "carry" this job. [...] Very often what we deal with is not life-threatening. [...] [Instead, patients in my specialty] have "functional" "expectation[s]," [...] and very often you have to think about things from their perspective [...]. I need to know what their jobs are. I need to be considerate of what they need to do for their jobs to have such "expectation[s]," and what I can do to help them. [...] If you always put yourself in a very superior position, you will never understand [patients' symptoms]. The more I have done, the longer I have worked, the more I feel that I need to think from their standpoint. So my contrasting view is that [...] the more experienced the [specialist doctor] is, the more you will forget that you are a doctor in this so-called "superior" position, and the more you will talk to "patient[s]" in a down-to-earth way. Only then can you help them. [CAN]

The first doctor quoted under the last theme also discussed humility in conjunction with empathy. He said:

> The longer you have worked, the cleverer you think you are [...] Your "knowledge" has started to "accumulate," and you'll think that what the "patient" has to say cannot compare with what you say. You will think, "You must listen to me. I am the 'authority.' You should do this this and this." Or perhaps you don't think of yourself as very clever. You might think of yourself as pitiful instead: "I was on 'call' yesterday, and it's very tough for me. Don't 'expect' me to give you any good 'service.'" But I always think that you must always, always, try to let go of your "ego," and what you yourself think is correct. [CAN]

A third doctor also talked about the importance of remaining grounded: "When I was a 'houseman,' someone once told me: 'Don't be a hero.' I agree, 'because I'm not trying to play God or be a hero by being a doctor' [ENG]. I think I'm just trying to help when I can. 'I need to show care for the patients' [ENG]" [CAN]. She discussed the need to always be on her guard to make sure that patients received the best care possible: "'I think you need to stay humble and modest no matter how many years of experience you have, which sometimes you forget' [ENG]."

2.3.2.6 Effectively Performing Non-Clinical Roles

As doctors progressed in their public hospital careers, they were assigned non-clinical duties alongside clinical ones. Some doctors saw the need for and the benefits of these duties to their clinical work and the healthcare system as a whole, and therefore looked beyond such non-clinical work as mere chores they were forced to do. One doctor said:

> I've been in this position, to which I was promoted, for two to three years now. [...] Right now I also need to do some "administrative" things, so I understand a bit more about what, in hospitals, apart from "clinical" operations, the "management"—that is supervisors—demand, or what their demands are when "run[ning]" a "specialty" or a "department." Because of this I can see in a more comprehensive way. Before, I could only "focus" on patients. Now, I can think a bit more beyond patients—[for instance,] when I prescribe this "treatment" or "management," what the effect on patients is, or whether hospital administration would have any "concern[s]." I've started to think more about these types of things [...] throughout these years. [CAN]

Another doctor discussed how she had started to think about the importance of an efficient and improved system:

> In the past two years, I've started to think more broadly about the whole "system." For instance, how can the "team['s]" operation within the department, the process, make better use of resources? For instance, for some people, do we have ways to enable them to use these "service[s]" better? Are there any "tools" that can help us? [...] I've worked for this long, and all along my focus had been a bit different. Previously, I wouldn't think about things in the "system." I would think that these things didn't have to do with me, and that all I needed to do was to do what was right in front of me well. But now, I've started to slowly think that a complete "system," a good "system," will in fact distribute resources better, so it's in fact helpful, and not just about how you treat a patient. [CAN]

A third doctor described seeing the need for such non-clinical duties and enjoying them as she advanced in her career, despite them taking up much of her time. Being a clinical doctor then also involved being a non-clinical multi-tasker:

> When you are junior, you could "focus" on some more "clinical" things, but when you become more and more senior, you have more and more "administrative" things [to do]. Especially in public hospitals there are many administrative things [to take care of], for instance organizing "roster[s]"—whom to allow to go on leave and who can't go on leave. These kinds of things we also need to handle. [...] But it's "okay." I quite "enjoy" it. When you distribute the work amongst colleagues, or sometimes nurses come and ask for help with material supplies, you will think it's quite interesting. [...] [You need to figure out] how to obtain resources. You need to write a lot. When people "complain," not about myself, but about our "junior[s]," we have to help them reply. There are many such things. You will discover that it is busy, but that, as a doctor, you can only do things well when you take up many roles and take care of many things at the same time. [CAN]

2.3.3 Work Problems in Public Hospitals

Although the doctors interviewed had so far chosen to remain working in the public sector, they also pointed out problems in this sector which made their work more difficult, or which diminished the meaning of their work. Often these were systemic problems that individual doctors did not have much power to change. For some doctors, such problems created possible reasons for switching over into private-sector work in future.

2.3.3.1 Enhanced Patient Support in Private Care

Two doctors indicated how in the private sector, doctors may possibly be able to help patients more or in better ways than in the public sector. One doctor said:

> "In terms of" really helping people, [...] I'm guessing that it [the private sector] may be about the same, but I have friends who've gone out into the "private" sector, and they actually think that it's only in the private sector that they can help patients. Of course you're talking about wealthy people, but in fact many people have bought "medical insurance" these days, and you don't need to be very wealthy to have "surgery" done outside. [CAN]

Another doctor said:

> Some colleagues have just gone out into the "private" sector, and they've told me that in fact you can also help people in the "private" sector. Because your clinic is less rushed, you can really talk to them "in depth," and you can understand their "background" more carefully, "rather than" just giving them medicine and letting them go. [CAN]

2.3.3.2 High Workload

Many doctors discussed the heavy workload they faced in public hospitals. There is some overlap between this theme and some of the themes under the group "personal problems caused by work" to follow below. The difference is in the emphasis here on heavy workload as a work and work-related performance problem, whereas the themes under the next group of "personal problems" emphasize the effects of these problems on other aspects of interviewees' personhood, such as their mental wellbeing and emotions.

This theme will first start with quotations discussing the heavy workload in public hospitals in general. It will then continue with the two subthemes on clinical and non-clinical workloads respectively.

One doctor explained such workload problems in detail:

> Over half of the classmates in my year have gone out into the "private" sector. There must be some problems. Throughout the learning process, you can hear us say that there will be people who can teach you and let you develop. You can do many things. This is the attitude that a young doctor should have, and what a young doctor should do. But you have to consider something more, which is that in public hospitals the patient load is very big. [...] You go to work at a particular time, [but] you don't know what time you get off work. In writing, they say it starts from 8 am, but in reality, when your supervisor comes in at 8 am, I may need to be there at 7:30 am, or for more complex patients I have to be already there at 7:15 am. In terms of the time of getting off work, when is [this]? You have many things within the "schedule" that in reality you have to do, but the "schedule" has not "schedule[d]" them as things to be done by you. The things within the "schedule" are more than the things you can normally "handle"—very often administrative work, or some "planning" work, or some "review[ing]" work, that is, work that is not written into a "schedule." Or you supervise some [...] more junior people, and after they are finished you have to help them further, and look at things again. No one has allocated such time for you, so it's your own time, the time after work hours. [CAN]

Another doctor explained how these workload problems got worse for him as his career progressed:

> Starting from 10 years ago till now, I've gotten busier and busier. The longer I work [...], the more you discover that the higher your position, the busier you are, because when you know more, it's not like jobs outside where [...] the higher your position, the more leisurely it becomes—this won't happen, especially in [my specialty]. The higher you are, the more experience you have, and the more you know, then in fact the busier you become, and the easier it becomes to be "call[ed]" back when you are "off duty" or when it's nighttime, because some complicated or "emergency" operations have to be done. [CAN]

A third doctor described how having more time with patients could make a big difference on their relationship with them:

> If you can have a lot of time to talk to patients, or a lot of time to explain things to them, then it might be different. But ultimately, we're so busy that we can't even finish all our work. [...] If you spend too much time, you won't be able to go home even at 8 or 9 pm, and your spouse will complain. [CAN]

A fourth doctor summarized the situation by stating that "the 'workload' at public hospitals 'test[s]' our 'EQ' to the utmost" [CAN]. A fifth doctor, who had also worked overseas, said: "just the responsibility and the workload that you have to carry in Hong Kong are significantly more burdensome in Hong Kong, compared to other countries."

The heavy workload could not generally be mitigated by opting for part-time work. The doctor quoted just now who remarked on the challenge that work demands placed on her EQ said: "If public hospitals could solve this 'workload' problem, it's in fact a very attractive profession, and perhaps not so many people would have the desire to leave. According to what I know, the structure at public hospitals is that they do not encourage female doctors to work 'part-time'" [CAN].

However, if doctors could be given the option to work part-time in public hospitals, the advantages of such work, including the deep meanings that it held for many interviewees, could lead to more staff staying on even if they could earn more working a similar number of hours in the private sector.

Demanding Clinical Workload

This subtheme continues on from such general descriptions of interviewees' heavy workload, focusing specifically on doctors' very demanding clinical workload and the repercussions of this on their clinical practice. For instance, consultation times needed to be kept extremely short. One doctor said:

> In public hospitals, if you're not seeing some special "high-risk case[s]" on which you have to spend a lot of time and effort, [...] you may really need to finish seeing a "case" in five minutes, because there are too many people outside waiting. So frankly speaking, [...] the only thing not good about public hospitals is that you don't have enough time. You always have very many "patient[s]." For "low-risk" patients, perhaps their feeling is: "Do you seem too perfunctory?" But in fact there's just no way. You have too many time constraints. [...] I want to spend more time to chat with them, but I can't do it. [...] And [people might think,] "Why do doctors always seem to be facing the computer, seem to be mechanistic?" Because we need to talk to patients, listen to what you say, "mark" down what you have said, and then my brain needs to analyze this, all at the same time. So it seems that we even have less "eye contact" when we see "low-risk case[s]." [CAN]

Another doctor said that the work environment made it almost impossible for doctors to treat their patients with more care:

> I feel that the longer you work, the more you reach a point where in fact I don't think that the Hong Kong health care system is very "favorable." I think it forces everyone to be like the doctor you [the interviewer] have just discussed [who did not say anything during an examination], especially in the public sector. Because you can "imagine" my spouse [who is also a doctor] [...]: she has to see 40 to 50 "patient[s]" in one "session," and one session

> has only three hours. You can try to do the division. You just don't know how to see patients like that. The whole situation doesn't "make sense." But you can see that in Hong Kong, the "system" is like that. You can't devote very much effort to every "patient." You just can't. If you do, you overrun into the afternoon, and the "patient[s]" in the queue will come out and shout and all that. So I think sometimes it's the social environment and the "system" that force doctors to become like that. [CAN]

Two doctors described how the workload made building rapport with patients very difficult. The first doctor said:

> It's very difficult to see "case[s]" again that you've handled before. For instance, I conduct [a specialist procedure] eight or nine times a day. But I also do rounds in wards for 20 patients. You do rounds, and then you go to the clinic. You have clinics in the morning and in the afternoon, or you have surgeries in the morning and surgeries in the afternoon. You can't possibly slot in seeing "case[s]" you treated yesterday. You can't even finish the work you already have. It's difficult to establish a relationship that is a bit more "personal." And sometimes when patients come back, they don't see you. In public hospitals, it's difficult. Unless you clearly write down and tell administrative staff to let them see you again the next time—but not all staff are willing to do this. If I see [patients] from before their surgery, I do the surgery, and when they come back for follow-up consultations it's me again who sees them, then the relationship would be better. In public hospitals, there are good and not-so -good things, and the fact that every time you see a different patient and it's difficult to build rapport with them is something not so good. [CAN]

Another doctor had similar concerns: "If your 'rapport' with patients is good, patients understand [when there are complications]. So what I think is even more unfortunate is that, because our 'workload' is just so very heavy—we need to see perhaps 50 patients in four hours—we have very little time to 'build up rapport'" [CAN].

Doctors in general described a system that was bursting at its seams, where they knew they could not provide the care they wanted. One doctor said: "Even as a fresh graduate, you are responsible for [...] maybe 20 patients, all under your own care. Some of them can be really ill and it's really all on your hands, right? So it was challenging, it was overwhelming at first." Another doctor said:

> I think that the public system has its own limitations, but it is needed. Its limitations everyone knows about: all "waiti...ng time[s]" are very long, the "patient load" is getting bigger and bigger—before it may have been 100%, but now it may be 120%, and it's getting more and more. But these people also need expertise the most. [CAN]

A third doctor also described some of the compromises that were necessary:

> We cannot do what they advocate overseas: sitting down and taking good care of [patients] on an emotional level. I think if you interview some very front-line doctors, you should be able to see the pressure. Even when their hearts are dedicated to the work, the system will lead to them not being able to do anything, because for instance when they tell you that today there are many people coming in for a follow-up consultation, if I want to do the best I can and for everything to be absolutely ideal, the "clinic" will not finish. [CAN]

However, such compromise may not be a long-term solution for some doctors, who may decide that they have no choice but to leave the public system, as we will later see in some of the themes under the group "personal problems caused by work."

Demanding Non-Clinical Workload

As mentioned, apart from clinical duties, doctors also had substantial non-clinical duties, which increased their overall workload. Although the doctors quoted under the theme of "effectively performing non-clinical roles" described these duties as beneficial to the workings of the system, and in one case as enjoyable, the two doctors quoted under this subtheme viewed their non-clinical workload less positively.

One doctor said:

> While I was "training," I didn't "expect" there to be these things. When you "envision" a doctor, you don't "envision" him or her doing office work, that is, doing "managerial" things. But "somehow" in "public hospital[s]," there is this "work" that needs to be done. "After all, we're working for a big organization" [ENG]. When we "run" a "department," you can't just go and treat people. [You need to make sure] the "equipment is there, and infection control" [ENG] "guidelines" need to be "update[d]." These things must be done, but not everyone likes doing these things. I don't mind doing them, but "I think it's starting to take up more time" [ENG]. [CAN]

Another doctor named some examples of such tasks, and the sense that they took valuable time away from his most essential duties. He said:

> We have to be responsible for "roster[ing]" so that colleagues can have "presentation[s]." We may have to see how many things we need to buy each year, and think about how to fill in "application form[s]" that "favor" us being able to buy these machines. And perhaps we have to go listen to some [talks on] the whole hospital's "infection control," and what we need to do. But perhaps this "infection control" has no direct relationship with [our specialty]. It is a meeting in the same place for all the "department[s]" together in the whole hospital. [...] But "as part of the whole team," we have to sit there for two to three hours to listen to such a meaningful talk on "Zoom." I think it's a pity, because when we take the time to do this thing, it will lead to us not having time for "training" or for surgeries. [CAN]

He contrasted the situation in Hong Kong with that in Singapore:

> Singapore has different "tracks." [...] There is a "stream" for doctors who specialize in "administrative" work. And then there's a specialized "clinical" "stream," where you only see patients and do surgeries. The third stream is in "research," that is you write "paper[s]" and "grant" [applications]. These three "stream[s]" are "independent," that is, you sign different "contract[s]" depending on which stream you choose. But "in Hong Kong, you only have one choice, which is to do everything" [ENG]. Not everyone is interested in all three things. So I think this is to me a bit of a "challenge," and also a "drawback." [CAN]

2.3.3.3 Dehumanization of Care

The heavy workload described can lead to problems not just for doctors' clinical practice, but also for patients who, because of it, may not be treated with careful consideration and respect. As we will see, this theme and the next theme of "departure from patient-centric care" are similar enough to be combined. However, we created this separate theme for the interview quotations where doctors themselves used such terms as "dehumanize" and "humane" that emphasized the stronger moral concern driving this theme. This is in contrast to the quotations in the next theme, which have a stronger focus on organizational governance.

One doctor said that when he was a "junior resident," he felt that:

> there's always pressure to try and create more room for the next patient, to discharge patients is as soon as feasible. I chose the word feasible over the word possible. [...] Many times, patients are good to leave, but then it's not feasible for them to, because there are just no outside community resources to take care of them—so [no] continuity of care. [...] But then there's that other pressure as well to see how I can make the next bed empty for the next patient to come in. So it seems quite Kafkaesque if you will, [...] in terms of just trying to get everything together and dehumanize the process, and just say: "Just try and get them well and get them out," and then the next patient comes in the next day and then you have... It's quite a Sisyphean or Kafkaesque... [...] There's always this trying to push the rock up the hill and then you're still not there.

Another doctor discussed how to overcome the systemic problems of overcrowding and long wait times:

> To be very honest, I can't think of any ways. The only thing we can do is to [perform surgery on] urgent cases, and not on non-urgent cases. But for those so-called non-urgent cases, it's in fact not very "fair." "From" their perspective, or "from" their "relatives'" perspective, of course they think it's not very "fair." If you look at my "patient[s]," with the entire "patient floor" comprising a few hundred "patient[s]" altogether, then there's no other way. I also think sometimes, some things are not very humane. But there's no other way when you think about the whole "pool." [CAN]

Another doctor recounted a case where a patient told her how:

> the nurses in the previous ward did not treat him like a human being, and how here, with us [in our ward], we do treat him like a human being. Even within public hospitals, it's possible to be in a ward where the "staff['s] "workload" is perhaps even higher than ours. So were there [issues] with the language used or with manoeuvres that were not done gently enough? Because he was quite thin and weak, so sometimes if you're a bit rougher in your manoeuvres, then maybe he would find it tough. But [...] perhaps he didn't have the courage, being a well-mannered person, to say anything when you caused him to feel pain. And then perhaps he had endured this for a long time, and felt wronged inside, and only talked about this to a healthcare worker he trusted. So when he said that the previous ward didn't treat him like... He was crying the whole time. So when he was talking to me his tears were falling: they did not treat him like a human being. [CAN]

She further explained:

> It may not have been the case that the healthcare worker was very "intentionally" wanting to "induce pain on" him. Perhaps it was just the workload she had. Perhaps everyone was laid down and had to have abdominal fluids drained in the ward, so of course that was how you drained the fluids, she thought—"Don't 'say' so much. This is the way it's done." But perhaps he thought that he was "being dehumanized." [CAN]

As a result of this feeling, the patient ended up not pursuing further treatment, leading to the interviewee's dismay and sadness. The doctor's insight from this was that:

> The decisions a patient makes might not only depend on his own desire to continue to battle illness. Of course I think he had definitely digested the "pros and cons"—he was an "educated" person—but another consideration was that he had to think about the healthcare

> workers that he might come into contact with, and whether they would aggravate his "suffering." For a patient with so many physical discomforts, he felt like a human ball [being passed around] once he was hospitalized. [...] He said he decided not to do it [pursue further treatment]. What he meant was that he didn't want to prolong his suffering. But I think this suffering may in fact at times be induced by medical staff. [CAN].

2.3.3.4 Departure from Patient-Centric Care

Closely related to the above theme were the conflicts some doctors saw between the patient-centric care that hospitals should ideally provide as public organizations, and how they saw patients being treated in reality. One doctor observed a disjunction between patient care in theory and what she called "the profession in practice":

> Before, I studied at "medical school" for so many years, and the emphasis was always on things that were very "patient-oriented," very "patient-centered." And this is the way it should be—I still believe this. But in reality, in the "profession in practice," this is part of the "concern," and not the full starting point. At times I even think this is not the "primary concern." This is disappointing to me. I don't know if this is something that is inevitable when you put the "profession" into "practice," or it's just what happens when you put it into the public system. [CAN]

She continued to discuss this discrepancy within the context of the HA, which juggles goals that may conflict:

> Although [the HA's] goal is not profit—so its goal has differences from that of a "business"— "somehow" it's a bit like an "NGO." Its goal is not to make money, but "somehow" it's for attaining certain goals, and those goals are not geared towards people. For instance, in a commercial organization, the goal is to make money, and this is very obvious. But in the "HA," even if the purpose is neither money nor people—I don't even know what their primary purpose is—but really it's for some numbers, some standards. These standards in fact do not necessarily directly reflect that your "patient care" is very good. That is, I don't know where the intelligence behind them lies. "Somehow" when you put the "profession" within such a framework, I think it will influence "patient care." It's not all bad, but "somehow" it will sometimes "deviate from" what you imagine, and won't take this as a priority. It is "more determined by" not necessarily "patient benefit," but an "organizational benefit." In the end, the "patient" is of course a "part" of what the "organization" "serve[s]"—you can't say that it doesn't do this at all—but it also partially "serve[s]" the "government," and "serve[s]" I don't know what other things. [CAN]

Two other doctors similarly mentioned issues with patient care due to systemic and organizational problems. One doctor said: "I feel very... honestly, quite upset because I think the system is not treating our patients well." Another doctor argued against the cold and calculating use of numbers:

> You calculate how much it costs for patients to stay there each day. But hey, if they need to stay, they need to stay. You wouldn't force them to stay. [...] If you need this much, then you need this much. [...] It shouldn't be the case [where we get asked], "Why did you use so much money for 'bed stay[s]'?" It shouldn't be like this. I need however much I need. [...] So many people can see these problems here. Essentially you spend a lot of effort to "treat" "patient[s]," but what they put importance on isn't this. They don't put importance on "clinical outcome." They put importance on the "number[s]" outcome. Hence many people have left. [CAN]

She also saw some projects that were imposed as taking away time and resources from patient care, and wanted the focus to be instead on the provision of new services that would truly benefit patients, in an interview quotation that resonates with the theme of "bureaucratic barriers" to follow below. She said:

> Those "project[s]" need a lot of time and staff, and waste a lot of the nurses' and the doctors' time. But if those "project[s]" are useful, I think it's "okay." But many "project[s]" aren't done with the "patient" in mind. They can be very useless things, for instance moving the patient's bedside file from paper form to some IT "iPad" form. This leads to a large number of "project[s]," "which doesn't really benefit the patient," right? It doesn't make any difference. But you spend a lot of time having meetings, a lot of time on how to "implement" this thing, and then nurses and "ward staff" don't focus on taking care of patients, but on where to put my "iPad," how to "set up" my "station" to charge, this kind of thing, "which" I think is very useless. When you "propose" something really useful, "for example" [a specialist procedure that is] "much more effective" [than procedures currently used], [...] this is really worth doing. Yet this cannot be implemented. Why? Because many parties say: "No. Why should this resource be given to your 'department' and not my 'department'? Then how about my 'department'?" So there are lots of such "interdepartmental" fights over things. Shouldn't this be coordinated by the "head office" of the "Hospital Authority"? Why else do we have the "HA"? [CAN]

She understood, but disagreed with, the reason behind IT measures being implemented over improved specialist procedures: "When you switch to these 'IT' things, it's fast—you get results fast, and can already do a lot. But if you really need to 'coordinate' a new [specialist] 'service,' you need a very long time. [...] So it's too 'bureaucratic'" [CAN].

2.3.3.5 Reduced Pay Relative to Private Practice

Doctors pointed out that private sector pay could exceed public sector pay for some specialties. One doctor pointed out that "a bunch of people have left, and there have been especially many [who have left] these past two years. Perhaps this is because they want to emigrate and they want to earn a sum of money outside, and then leave" [CAN]. But even before this, "many people had in fact already left. Of course, the difference between pay in the 'private' versus the 'public' sector is really very big" [CAN]. Another doctor said: "Why do our colleagues leave? It's very practical. They have to face financial pressures. You could say that doctors earn a lot, but they might have to spend a lot on sustaining their family" [CAN]. A third doctor pointed to what she saw as a generational shift in thinking about money-making:

> Many "junior doctor[s]" these past few years have been wanting to go out into the beauty health sector to earn money: injecting "Botox," and using laser to remove pigment spots. [...] In that "generation," the firmness of will, to me, seems to be weaker and weaker. But conversely, they are very clear in their goals, that is, they won't waste time. They think that since after they pass their "specialist" exams, in the end, they will go out into the private sector and work in a more profitable business anyway, so why not go out to "develop" their "career" earlier? I think this also makes sense. [CAN]

2.3.3.6 Bureaucratic Barriers

Public hospitals are governed by administrative and organizational rules and regulations. Some doctors commented on the restrictions that these could pose to their work. One doctor discussed how this could push doctors to leave the public sector:

> Public hospitals have many limitations. We do our best to push for [more resources]. It's true that some colleagues feel like they've had enough, [for instance when] in public hospitals there isn't this particular service, or they wish to push that particular service but it's very difficult. So they go out [into the private sector].
>
> It's funny: in public-sector organizations, specialists can in theory pursue further study overseas after completing their training. Often, when doing further study, you don't learn about some existing services—[the goal is] to learn some new service and bring it back to Hong Kong. But when you want to start these services and it's one difficulty after another, then this is a very big inducement—that's why middle level colleagues, after completing training, will leave. [CAN]

Another doctor said: "Of course, if you ask if everything is very rosy, then of course it's not": his workplace "is a very bureaucratic place, and sometimes such bureaucracy rather ties you down" [CAN]. A third doctor also thought the system was "too bureaucratic," and that "that's why many people have left," and not "because working for the HA is tough" [CAN].

One doctor discussed the possible mismatch between roles that suited people's abilities as opposed to roles that they were assigned by the system, creating restrictions that can wear doctors down. She said:

> Ultimately, public sector organizations have public sector organization problems, and they need to, and like to, find some people who can develop within the system. So this is different from private organizations. Private organizations very often suit people who can develop something they like and are suited to doing to the best, and then your whole organization will improve as a whole. But public sector organizations are not like this, do not run like this. They will say to senior people: since you have this rank, you go do administrative work. But maybe that senior person who got promoted does not like doing administrative work, but likes seeing patients. Then they say "No. You should try your best to do more administrative work, because people in your position need to do administrative work." But some junior people may like doing administrative work, but [they say] "You're so junior—why should you do administrative work? Administrative work involves calling the shots." So things are not within your own control. [CAN]

She used another example, that of teaching, to illustrate her viewpoint on the restrictions of the bureaucracy of public sector organizations like the HA:

> Let's say I like teaching. Teaching is something that the Hospital Authority sees as something extra, that is something outside of services. So teaching is of course good, but you use your own time. For instance, if I develop something new, then of course I want other people at other hospitals to know about this new thing. If they don't know about it, [and] I want to go to other hospitals to teach people how to do it, then because you belong to this hospital, you can't go to other hospitals to do things, [so you can't]. So there are lots of restrictions. [CAN]

2.3.3.7 Teamwork Challenges

Although teamwork was discussed as an advantage to working in public hospitals under the category of "work benefits" earlier, teamwork could also cause friction and pose problems for effective work. One doctor said:

> Because in public hospitals, we very much emphasize "teamwork" for many things, if a "junior" or someone else does something wrong, affecting the patient, your whole "team" is responsible. So poor "outcome[s]" will affect you. You will work more carefully, hoping that the "junior[s]" or others [...] in your "team," can work together and be more careful with "patient care." Of course as a "team," we have to take "feedback," and look back at our results. Only then can our methods improve. [CAN]

Several doctors talked about potential discontent with uneven workload distribution amongst team members. One doctor said:

> Between different 'specialt[ies'] work, there is some unfairness [in workload distribution]. The HA often has the same pay for different amounts of work. Very often work is not distributed evenly. You're bound to have this within a very big organization. But after you "recognize" these things, you discover that these things aren't that important, and that it's just some "noise." "At the end of the day," you want to help "patient[s]." You will see clearly that being very frustrated and agitated is meaningless, so you just drop those things. [...] You do the best you can with things "within" your "control." [...] As you work longer and longer, you see through things and accept them. If not, you will just leave. [CAN]

Another doctor cited this as a possible reason why some people left: "I guess some people feel like they're getting paid proportional to their effort [in the private sector], and people might feel that's fairer, because in our system some people do more, some people do less, and you get paid the same" [CAN].

Finally, one doctor described an instance—which made a lasting impact on her—when teamwork broke down. She recounted being verbally "torn into" by a senior doctor when she was still learning the ropes of her specialty:

> I didn't know how to do something, so I asked the nurses, who I think taught me the wrong way. I couldn't do it, so [the senior doctor] shouted at me: "You don't know how to do this, but you don't even ask." I remember thinking: "How would I dare ask you if you shout at me like this, even if I don't know how to do it?" [CAN]

Because of this incident, she resolved herself to "never cause people to not even dare to ask me something" [CAN].

2.3.3.8 Workforce Shortage

Several doctors discussed serious staff shortages, and how this impacted their work. One doctor said:

> You become more familiar with the process, so you can fly through things a lot more quickly, but more workforce shortage is definitely a problem. Just as an example, my team in my hospital [...] had 6.5 doctors two years ago, and now we're down to 3.5, and that makes a big difference. And the number of patients is not really going down, and we're getting a lot more patients. It's difficult to handle.

However, he felt compelled to stay because "if you leave, then you bring the whole team with you, and then what? I don't know what they would do." He also thought there was a lack of "long-term planning"; instead, "it's all just kind of stop gap." His wish was that in a few years' time, "if I'm still in the public sector, [...] our team can grow to a to a reasonable number where we can handle cases reasonably quickly and efficiently." Another doctor also said the number of doctors was not keeping up with the increase in patients: "There are more and more patients, and the number and experience of doctors are comparatively insufficient" [CAN].

Other doctors discussed the difficulties in having the next generation of doctors trained because of a lack of doctors of a suitable rank. One doctor said:

> Within the Hospital Authority, how to "retain" some mid-rank people is currently quite challenging. You can say that there's a chance that there will be a gap in the ranks. [...] Many mid-rank people have already left, and this is excluding the issue of emigration. [...] Before, our seniors [...] could very quickly not have to do some things themselves. But now, you discover that 20 years ago you were helping juniors, and 20 years later you are still helping those very junior [doctors], because the mid-rank people have left. This is a problem. [CAN]

Another doctor said that because of the "personnel gap" due to people leaving, she covered the duties of staff with experience spanning across 10 years:

> Within, above, and below [my rank], there is no one, so I'm the representative of this span of 10 years' [experience]. So people [ranking] above me ask me to do things to help them, and colleagues [ranking] below me also ask me. I'm doing things that are the most front-line, but I also do logistical things. All work duties "overlap" and are draped over my shoulders. I don't even know what my upcoming "duties" are, because I'm almost like a "relieving" worker, that is, I go wherever there are not enough people. [CAN]

A third doctor said:

> "There's an imbalance between the number of trainers and trainees. [...] [Being] trainees means that they are not independent. They still need to rely on the supervisor. Trainers are [people] who have finished training for at least two years. We only have nine trainers at the moment, so every trainer has to take up more than two trainees—on average 2.1 trainees." [ENG; these sentences were in English although the interview was mainly in Cantonese]. In terms of the "training," this is not a good thing, and for the trainer, it is very demanding. Compared with 10 years ago, the ratio was perhaps one to one, but now it's one to two, "so you can imagine the quality of the training would be very different." Before, performing a surgery, I can teach you to do the entire surgery. But now, perhaps I need to show you the first half, "and then the other trainee has to look at the other half," so everyone's share has been divided up by half. So the "quality" of this "training" is not the same, but [our specialty's] "training" period has not increased. It's still six years. In six years' time, I have to make a person who cannot at all examine [a particular organ] into someone who knows how to do everything, from examinations to surgery, by herself. This amount of time in fact is very little. [CAN]

A fourth doctor said:

> There have been too many people leaving, and all of them have been mid-rank people. [...] This group of 30- to 40-year olds have the most duties. [...] You have just reached the stage when you are handling a large "number" [of cases], [...] so you have significant "experience" to teach people below you. But right now, in the middle ranks, lots of people have left, so some "service[s]" cannot in fact be "continue[d]." This is a very big problem. [CAN]

She expanded on the seriousness of this issue:

> In fact, the "plastic surgery service[s]" at some centres are not able to "continue"; "head and neck service[s]" are not able to "continue"; "breast surgery service[s]" are not able to "continue." The result is that after the people who were there have all left, you cannot "train" people below them [...]. The trainees who are left have just graduated, and cannot be "train[ed]" on time before [people] retire. The ones in the middle have all gone. So what can you do? [CAN]

2.3.3.9 Restricted Career Progression

Although, as described under the theme "further training and enhanced learning," numerous doctors thought that working in public hospitals gave them more development opportunities than the private sector would, some doctors also described headwinds in further career development in the public sector. One doctor said: "Many people don't manage to get a promotion, and remain in the same position for a long time, so they want to go out and change their environment" [CAN]. Another doctor said that some doctors "think that they aren't really able to get what they want." The situation in "every 'unit' or 'specialty' is different. In some specialties [...], they get promoted very quickly. In [other specialties], they get promoted relatively slowly. So if some of your classmates have already been promoted very rapidly, but you are still in the same place, then you'll be unhappy, and will leave" [CAN]. This, as a third doctor pointed out, could become a staff retention issue. She emphasized how important it was to retain these doctors, since "it takes eight, nine years, or even more than that, after your graduation to reach this status [of subspecialization after initial specialization]" [ENG; this sentence was in English in a mainly Cantonese interview]. If "they think they can't develop anything further," and "they put a lot of effort in their work" but this is "not valued," with the emphasis instead placed on such things as "making the numbers look better, that is, how many days it takes to 'discharge' people" [CAN], then people might choose to leave.

Promotional criteria may also not be related to work performance, but on vacancies. One doctor discussed factors pushing doctors to leave the public sector:

> The first is the issue of recognition, because promotion in public hospitals... [does not necessarily depend on] how good you are at doing work, or how successful you are, or how many people you've saved—they don't look at such things. Rather they look at how many people have left, and how many "consultant[s]" your department should have according to the rules, and how many "associate consultant[s]." This has been set. If no one leaves, there will be no vacancies, no matter how successful you are. If you like staying at your hospital, you won't have promotion opportunities. This is a problem with the system. [CAN]

This is in contrast to the work recognition doctors might be accorded outside of public hospitals:

> When you go on "international" exchange, you'll discover that you are not so bad on the international stage, that you are recognized internationally. [...] Some of the things you do are quite "high-end." Even some more senior people will [say]: "Come and teach here. You don't need to learn anything, just come and teach and have fun." This international

recognition is something that I think the HA cannot give you. So this becomes an even greater impetus to try "academic" [work]. Will you be able to help even more patients at this higher and broader level? [CAN].

Finally, one doctor mentioned the problem of hindrances in further development, but saw them as part of problems that each system had. She said that although people may leave because "they think that they can't develop because they are constrained by the system,"

That's not how I see it, because I think no matter which "system" you are in, it will have its "limitations." In the "HA," these are the "patient load" and "waiting time[s]," which affect your "management." But the "private" system is similarly "affected by" the "cost," which affects your "management," because not every "patient" can spend such money to treat their illnesses. [CAN]

2.3.3.10 Resource Allocation Challenges

This theme is related to the previous ones of "high workload" and "workforce shortage," but goes beyond workload and workforce shortage issues in outlining the effects of insufficient resources and capacity. For instance, two doctors discussed the resource allocation problems that advances in clinical treatments—otherwise a positive development—had caused. One doctor said:

The number of investigations and treatments we can order keeps increasing. This sounds good, but if you can arrange all of these, you will need to read more and more reports, and think about more and more things. Previously, a type of "lung cancer" would be terminal. 10 years ago, there was new "targeted therapy." This year, it's different. There are more and more types of targeted therapy. [...] For the patient it's a good thing, but for the doctor, the source of stress is that you have to finish everything you can arrange for [the patient] within a limited "consultation time." [...] Previously 10 patients could be seen in one session, so why can't you see 10 patients now? But even if I could, I still need to use more time to see them, because the things I need to discuss, and need to check, have become more and more. [...] So I think one very big "limitation" is that as the number of patients increases, although our resources have increased, what we "offer" patients has also increased, but it leads to us finding it more stressful to explain and arrange treatment options, to arrange "follow-up," and so on. I think these things are difficult, but there haven't been many extra resources put in, or extra capacity given to us. It's not just simply a workforce shortage issue—it's a "capacity" issue. [CAN]

Another doctor similarly thought:

I think patients' demands on us have increased. I'm not using [the word] "demand" [CAN] as a negative "term," but purely to say that physically and medically, their demands on us have genuinely increased, because illnesses have become more complicated. [...] Some diseases couldn't be treated before, and you would see them and say that they couldn't be treated and say goodbye, but now you can't just let them go, because many things have become treatable. So it's that "triad" [...]: "cost, time," and "quality." It's difficult to do all three things very well, that is, you want low cost without waiting times, and very good "quality". At this point, we can't see this "perfect triad" happening. [CAN]

Other doctors discussed the long wait times and the potential repercussions for patients. One doctor said:

> There are different scans [and] different investigations that we have to arrange for the patients, and there's a huge wait[list] that's not reasonable at all. I mean, if you have a lung mass and I'm trying to book a CT [scan] for you, and they give me an appointment [in three years], you'll be long dead by that time. It is frustrating. [...] They keep talking about it, but [...] the problem boils down to the load of patients. [...] And this is only going to increase; it's not going to come down. [...] It's a really tough job to solve this problem, but I don't think we're really doing much about it right now.

Another interviewee expressed how powerless doctors were to change this situation, and how frustrating it was to be confronted by patients about it:

> Our queue for surgeries in particular is very long. So even when we really want to help some patients, it's a bit impossible to. [...] The patient comes in, and it's as if we're fighting. They complain: "Why does it take so long?" But in fact we can't solve systemic problems. [CAN]

2.3.4 Personal Problems Caused by Work

The previous group identified interview themes on work problems for public hospital doctors without covering the scope of personal problems and doubts that work could cause. This group contains themes on these, which cover topics ranging from the impact on doctors' emotions and personal lives, to their internal struggles as they faced work that fell short of the values they had imbued it with.

2.3.4.1 Disillusionment

As their careers progressed, some doctors felt that the ideals and meanings they wanted to endow their work with became diminished, either temporarily or permanently. One doctor, for instance, said: "Before, I became a bit lost as I worked. It wasn't 'exactly' that I didn't know whether to be in [my specialty]. I just felt that the 'workload' was too 'heavy,' and I felt that it was eroding my willpower. That is, that passion—it was being a bit eroded" [CAN]. Another doctor also described how the gap between her ideal conception of the work, and the reality of it, had grown bigger over time:

> The way the public thinks of this profession—that is, what I have heard other people say is their view of this profession—comes close to the way I also thought about it before: that is, that people [in it] should be very "high-end," very "proper," very "decent," having "goodwill," having a lot of "faith," [...] having very "high moral standard[s]." So perhaps the "picture" was very "ideal." And I thought everything would be very "patient-oriented." [...] But now I don't necessarily see it in these ways. [...] Whatever [people's] line of work is doesn't really "define" them. You can't say that because they're doing this line of work, that they are the ways that I just described. [...] To put it simply, if I have to be more honest, I don't see these people in such an "ideal," perfect way. [CAN]

This could be seen as part and parcel of coming face-to-face with the realities of work. But if the extent of disillusionment is too great, it can have a big negative impact on doctor's happiness with their work as their career progresses:

> If you ask "junior doctor[s]" right now, and they haven't left for the private sector, one reason is of course that they don't have a professional qualification yet. But strictly speaking, if you really want to leave, then you don't even need to work for the "HA" for your first year—you can go out and be a "GP." But if you ask some "junior[s]," I think their willingness to stay is high, because "somehow" it's not been so eroded, so "blunt[ed]." But the "senior" people, some will have been "blunt[ed]," and one of the reasons is because the work is "demoraliz[ing]." [CAN]

One doctor also mentioned how the HA's lack of accommodation of doctors' different needs as they entered different stages in their lives meant that staying in a public hospital role could become untenable:

> When you work until you marry and have children, you again think about how much time you should spend on work. It's already no longer that type of "idealistic" and "naïve" feeling of needing to help others. You start to have "practical issues" you need to think about. Many female doctors in public hospitals, when they start to marry and have children, waver at that point, because the HA is not "part-time friendly." So maybe people would rather go out into "part-time" work in the "private" sector, and their "part-time salary" would already be equal to the "full-time" "HA" salary. [CAN]

One interviewee objected not to the workload she had to face, but to what the workload meant for the satisfaction she could get from their work:

> Throughout, the thing I have liked the most is seeing patients. This is the thing that gives me the most "satisfaction." So when it gets very busy, and we can't spend time on patients, for some doctors, that is those who like front-line medical work, the satisfaction is very low. I've heard of many people leaving public hospitals because of such reasons. [CAN]

Finally, one interviewee felt so disillusioned about the insurmountable problems she had identified in public hospital work that she could not think of what to say to persuade others to stay. She said: "I myself no longer 'believe in' this. I think that when you reach a stage where you can't take it anymore, you need to leave. I need to take care of my 'personal mental health.' I can't go to work every day this 'frustrated'" [CAN]. Like the interviewees quoted before, she contrasted this with how she felt when she first started off in her career:

> When I graduated, I thought my future was bright. [...] You thought that you would have many "opportunities," that you would learn all kinds of things, and that many people could teach you. You would have many opportunities to "develop" things. This was the way I viewed everything when I graduated. All resources seemed very sufficient, with resources not just referring to money or facilities—those aren't the biggest problems. Right now, the biggest problem is [a lack of] "manpower." The difference is really too big. [CAN]

2.3.4.2 Psychological Impact of Losing Patients

When patients' treatments resulted in bad outcomes instead of recovery, doctors' mental state could be seriously affected. One doctor described it as "quite 'traumatic,'" and "any deaths" as "quite big trauma for the entire team and for individual doctors" [CAN]. Unanticipated poor outcomes could be particularly difficult to deal with:

When it's due to a disease you can't treat, that's different, but if it's "unexpected," and you find out that the final "outcome" is that you can't save [the patient], then you will be very despondent. So how to get out of that? The only thing to do is for everyone to review [what happened], and then to be more careful the second time. I'm not saying that it's [always] due to mistakes, but sometimes, for some things, you can't predict everything, and even if you try your hardest, you may not be able to help. This is not something that can be helped. [CAN]

Another reason for a deep emotional impact arising from patient death comes from "treating [patients] over a long period of time," and "establishing a long-term relationship with them":

For those cases, you feel sad not because you didn't do well, but because you've treated this patient for so long, and you hope that you can help them, but in the end you can't. For instance, some patients who have a blocked bile duct [...] wait for a liver transplant but they can't wait any longer, and in the end they don't make it. This will make you feel very despondent. So there are different levels that can affect your emotions. [CAN]

A second doctor described how he needed to learn to cope with the emotional fallout of patient complications. He said:

There was a period of time when I was very "down," especially in the first few years after I returned to Hong Kong from "training" [overseas], [when] I started to handle very complex and difficult cases. There were cases with complications. [...] For some time I would find it difficult to overcome [these emotions]. Luckily [...] the passage of time helps. And I think sometimes we have good supervisors who will comfort you. I think slowly as time passes it becomes better. [...] People used to say it all the time: behind every prominent doctor there is a line of, a group of, souls who follow them. [...] Every case that I cannot save is unforgettable to me. Patients who have complications make a deep impression on me. [CAN]

Recounting two such cases, he said:

[The first case] went to court and it dragged on for a long time. At the time I cried for a long time. I thought, [...] why couldn't I do anything? [...] And then when I was older, there was another time at [another hospital]. [...] Because [the patient] was young, and perhaps because we didn't communicate well enough, her family again complained to the utmost, to the extent where we had to have a "board" [to handle the case]. I sat there, and of course it was not a happy experience. I was surrounded by family members who criticized me for around an hour. [CAN]

Although he had learned to cope, these patients still left their mark on him:

If you ask me about what has left a deep impression on me, they're the patients I could not save, or [for whom] complications arose during surgery, or in these past few years one or two cases who because of complications [...] could not be saved. Those leave a deep impression on me. I always remember them. It's like they've been stamped onto my heart. Performing high-risk surgeries is bound to give rise to such situations. [CAN]

2.3.4.3 Physical and Mental Exhaustion

Although the doctors interviewed could all cope with the demands of their work, for instance through the strategies described in the next group of themes, the working conditions described under the previous group led to some doctors' ongoing physical and mental exhaustion. One doctor, whose entire interview was otherwise a description of her full dedication to her work, said:

> When do I waver [in the resolve to stay in the public system]? When I'm really too busy, and think that it's really tough, so tough that I feel there's no "support," or sometimes... I think the most "frustrat[ing]" is when sometimes, when many private doctors "refer" some very difficult "case[s]" here, and you can feel that the "patient" is very "helpless." And then it's as if you have to shoulder the entire responsibility in overseeing such a "difficult" case. At such a time, [...], you think it's really very difficult, it's very tough. Why do you have so many cases that you need to handle simultaneously? You are working so hard that you're being worked to the bone. And as I mentioned, I'm interested in everything, so [...] I need to do "clinical" things, and then "admin[istrative]" things, and then "academic" things. When everything is chasing after me, then at that point when my pressure levels become very high, sometimes I really would think, "Hey, if you go out to the 'private' sector, it will be simpler. It won't be so tough, and you can treat only 'low-risk case[s].'" This of course "deviat[es]" from my own value system. But when you want to be able to breathe, you may waver. But "otherwise," I think for now my sense of satisfaction is higher staying in public hospitals and teaching hospitals. [CAN].

Another doctor said:

> I've been working here for over 10 years, and have started to see and experience the internal problems of public hospitals, whether it's the organizational structure of medical care, or the [...] approach to handling the problem of "clustering." The workload, with relatively little support, and always a lack of staff; the pull of the private sector: of course [these things] will make you start to feel a bit enervated working in the public system. You'll feel that you don't know why you're working yourself to the bone. The purpose becomes blurry. So many friends have left because of this for private organizations. [CAN]

He elaborated:

> I hear of many colleagues suffering from "burnout" in public hospitals. This includes myself. I have also suffered from "burnout" before. I felt it was really very hard going, and I needed to take a week to rest. Working till I suffered from burnout in a public hospital was because I felt like I was not having much of a "life," that is, my "work-life balance" had become completely "distort[ed]." I would be constantly "call[ed]" back and work. After work I would return home to sleep. [CAN]

A third doctor repeatedly expressed his sense of feeling crushed throughout the interview. He said:

> You just feel defeated sometimes, to be honest. I always struggle to eat during work, but today I haven't eaten at all and this is not abnormal. But I just feel that if I've been working in the same place for 10 years, I should be able to get some regular meals as a minimum, right?

In a view that falls to some extent under the scope of the previous theme of "restricted career progression," he expressed his uncertainty that conditions would improve with career advancement:

> Most of our bosses [...] will be telling us how they have been through the same hardship when they were young, but they would be doing it for maybe one or two years, and they would be promoted to a position where you don't have to go through these kinds of hardships, right?

> Whereas for doctors nowadays, the room for promotion is very limited, and you have to go through these kinds of hardships for a way longer period. And that's defeating sometimes.

He had not yet left the public sector, partially for reasons unknown to himself, and partially because he felt he owed an obligation to his team members. He described his spouse asking him: "Why are you doing this?," and being unable to come up with a response: "I really don't know what to tell her." Whereas the earlier theme of "feeling indispensable" was a value from which doctors derived positive meaning, and a productive reason for staying in public hospital work, for this doctor, feeling indispensable forced him to stay in his work, rather than him wanting to: "If I bail out, [...] how will the team cope with it? [...] I think if I leave, the other members will also follow suit and pretty much the team will collapse or disappear. [...] I don't want to be the one that proves the trigger [for an exodus]." He explained that "we do talk about stuff like that in our team and say: 'Hey, if you're going, you better let me know earlier, right? We're going to jump together.' It's kind of sad that that's what's holding us together."

A fourth doctor, who conveyed throughout the interview how much she loved her public hospital work, said:

> If I think that I'm being so much affected by my work, that my "workload" is so heavy, that I'm having "physical" or other health problems, perhaps this would "push" me towards leaving public hospitals, because I wouldn't be able to "handle" it anymore. I know [...] some doctors younger than me who told me that within their circles of surgeons, a few had developed kidney stones. [...] Within [our specialty], even some [doctors] who only see cases [and do not have to perform procedures] feel "guilty" about going to the toilet, let alone surgeons, who entirely don't have the chance to go to the toilet. [At least] we have the chance to go [to the toilet], but it's just that we have so many cases. [CAN]

Her workload was her main source of continuing anxiety:

> Working at the public hospital, the thing that can really get me down is [whether I have] the ability to see how many cases within an hour. This can really bring out my "stress level[s]." [...] I surreptitiously think, "Am I being fast enough in seeing cases?" This kind of "stress" [...] for me is a negative "stress." [CAN]

Although she had learned how not to have her emotions affected for too long by problems with patients, she was still trying to cope with the negative effects of the workload on her mental wellbeing:

> Right now, although I'm not being affected by "patients' negative emotion[s]," I am being affected by "negative emotion[s]" deriving from work stress, because I'm not yet able to "handle" this as well as I want. When I go to work and I'm very busy, my "EQ" starts to become lower. [...] Because work hours are too long, we cannot "physically" "recover." When we don't sleep enough, our mental state becomes strained, or the way we think is not clear enough, so our emotional state will also be a bit poorer. [CAN]

This had made her "feel lost before. I think this was last year, when because my 'workload' was sometimes so heavy, I thought that at times I almost couldn't 'handle' it" [CAN]. Although she was managing at the time of the interview, "Because [the workload] is just too much, I think being 'part-time,' I could 'handle' that type of 'stress level' more easily" [CAN], although, as she pointed out, going part-time was not an option the HA commonly offered to its doctors.

Two other doctors described the consequence of feeling drained on their medical practice. One doctor said:

> For some things, [...] if I have more time, I can ask questions in more depth, and I can offer even better advice. But on the one hand are time constraints, and on the other hand, I think when you are very busy, we as doctors don't have the mental strength to do these things. That is, you yourself don't want to ask further questions. [...] When you're very tired, very busy, then in fact, when you reach a certain level, it directly affects the quality. [...] Before, I would not pay much attention to myself being in such a state. I just felt I had to keep working, keep working, keep working. But I just felt I couldn't achieve as much as I wanted, [...] that things just didn't reach the desired place. You put in a lot of effort, but there is just something missing. And then I gradually "reflect[ed] on" and paid attention to when this would happen more often, and I discovered it was when I was very busy. I think my brain would not "run" very well when I was tired. [CAN]

Another doctor said:

> It's really very tough, because it's very "mentally challenging," and the "responsibility" is very big. When you're very tired you will start to lose some of your own very important "value[s]." For instance, you will become angry very easily, lash out at others very easily, you won't want to continue, and you'll think "Let's just not do such a good job. Let's not give the patient 100% of my effort." I think all public hospital doctors are facing these things. [CAN]

Two additional doctors described their sense of dejection at patients' complaints about hospital conditions that they had no control over. One doctor said:

> I've experienced being complained about, being asked "Why do you need to operate on me after having been 'on call' for 24 hours? Why can't they find a doctor who is more alert to do the operation?" [Or] being asked why operating theater [surgeries] kept being "delay[ed]" due to "COVID." [...] I understand [patients'] concerns, and understand that they've been waiting for a long time. Sometimes when I hear these things I get very discouraged. [CAN]

Another doctor said:

> You can save some people, but never all. And in some cases, you've tried your best and there's nothing else you can do. But many people think that not being able to save someone means a medical mistake. And then you'll be under a lot of pressure, and they will lodge many complaints about you. So it's a bit depressing. Because think about it: in the private sector, they usually do some simple... that is, complex [procedures] will be left to us. If you don't do them, they will die, but if you do them, they may not live either. If they're done and the "outcome" is not good, they will think medical mistakes have been made. [CAN]

2.3.4.4 Challenges Balancing Work and Personal Life

Because of their workload, doctors could find it difficult to attain even a semblance of work-life balance, with competing demands placing a strain on aspects of their lives outside of work, although they also explained that this did not negate the meaning of their work to them. One doctor said:

> I could at midnight have to return to hospital to handle something that other people can't handle. [...] Because the "case[s]" we handle are too "rare" and too complex, on "public holiday[s]," on lunar new year day, we don't go for new year visits or anything. When I was a bit younger I didn't go for lunar new year visits, but had to rush back to the hospital, because I had to do some special "procedure[s]." If these weren't done the [patient] would definitely die. So it's very stressful, but you'll discover that yes, it's very "stressful" and very tough, but it's something meaningful. [CAN]

Another doctor said: "it's tough for us right now. For instance, [to provide a specific type of operation] around the clock, in one month, you need to work overnight for four to five nights" [CAN] to treat emergency cases. He did not feel it was possible to devote even more of his own time to provide better service:

> If you really want to provide service to the level of the private sector, then it's really tough. That is, seeing your patient after surgery is something that should happen, but perhaps your family will complain. We, the doctors who can conduct [this specialist procedure] independently, have been leaving [the public sector], and there are only four or five of us left. [...] So it's tough. Sometimes you need to get up at 2 or 3 am. So often you get up and your spouse doesn't even see you because you've already gone to the hospital. [CAN]

This detrimental work-life balance meant that working in public hospitals could be especially hard for parenthood, which could prove the catalyst for moving away from the public sector, as several doctors explained. One doctor said:

> Many people at my age have a "family." In particular, when female colleagues have children to take care of, they start having some "concern[s]" [about] whether they still have to be "on call" every day. Because we still use the system of having 5.5 working days a week, so sometimes we have to come back even in the weekend to work for half a day. So indeed a "portion" of colleagues have quit for these reasons. [CAN]

Another doctor said:

> The majority of people in my year have become mothers, and want to "quit" because of this reason: because they're not encouraged to work "part-time." So if they go "part-time," and in the private system can earn even more, and perhaps—and this we'd need to ask them—if the satisfaction from being a doctor is the same in the private sector, [...] then I think they will be find even less of a reason to stay. [CAN]

A third doctor with young children faced precisely this predicament. Since working at public hospitals "is of course tougher, with longer work times, and less flexibility," she said:

> Sometimes I think about whether time demands in the "private" sector will be more "flexible," so that I can strike a balance between my work and my life. I could spend more time doing my own things, or handling family things. And of course the money side is more attractive. Or perhaps in the "private" sector, although time demands are more "flexible," I can earn even more. I have considered these things. [CAN]

She elaborated at length on how parenthood affected the importance she placed on work-life balance, moving constantly back and forth in her discussion as she considered her conflicting options:

I think if I didn't have a "family," I may not consider the private sector. [...] But "as a woman and as a mother" [...], "I think there are more things to consider than just my career" [ENG]. [...] I think it's really difficult, to be honest. "I don't have a conclusion" [ENG]. [...] My "hours" are long. "I get up at 6 or 7, and by the time I get home" [ENG], I can't see my children. I "spend half an hour with them and I'm off to work" [ENG]. [...] You feel like you "miss out" on a "part of" their "lives."

"I think" it's a "work in progress," "because I'm coming to realize" [ENG]... Before, I was always "I'm all for it" [ENG]. Whatever you told me to do, "if I can do it, I'm saying yes" [ENG]. "I felt like I could do everything before" [ENG]. But "more recently," now that I have a "family," I think: "Oh, maybe I can't sacrifice that much" [ENG].

"I don't think there is an answer to it, and unfortunately... I read this article before" [ENG] [...] about "working moms," and it also said that, although there are many "high-powered women," they really "sacrifice" a lot of things. Its main point was that although men also obviously love their own children—I have many colleagues with young children [...]—it is "not that they don't want more time with them," but the whole "society" is "built up" in the way that from when you are little to when you grow up, a "mum is more of a child-caring role." "You will feel the burden that is expected of you." [...] If you can't do it you'll feel "mom guilt." I don't think it can ever be "g[otten] rid of." "Not that I'm quitting my job": "I think I'm at the stage where" I have to think about whether there must be some give-and-take. "Either I stick with some things at work," but "in that way" I think "it's maybe unfair to some of my colleagues" [ENG]. "Everyone's earning the same salary in public hospitals," so why do some people have to do more, some people less, some people "sacrifice" more, and some people work for longer periods? Some people don't mind. But "I will feel a bit of mom guilt if I don't put in more time at home." "But then I'll also feel [bad] if I don't put in as much as I can at work." "It's just something that you can't balance, and [in] public hospitals, unfortunately, if you work in the same department, you're getting the same pay." [...] Some "colleagues" "are more chill," and really don't do much of anything, and are more "hands-off at work." [...] But I don't want to be like this. "Just like" how some mothers are more "hands-off," and "leave their children to helpers or" get family members to take care of them, and don't think this is a problem "as long as they are safe." But I don't want it to be this way. "So I think it's difficult to be a very present mom and you want to have a very strong career at a public hospital. I find it difficult." [CAN]

2.3.4.5 The Risks of Complacency

Doctors discussed one danger to the meanings and values they ascribed to their work that feeling excessively worn out by their work could pose: of becoming complacent in their work, and performing it purely mechanically. Some of the quotations under this theme follow on from the theme of "disillusionment" earlier, and discussed this attitude as a possible specific *result* of the disillusionment that they mentioned. Other doctors did not reference the stage of disillusionment, instead describing their awareness of the risks of lacklustre work.

One doctor said:

You reach a point where I suddenly think that work that is relatively sacred turns into just another ordinary job. So everyone thinks: "I'm just doing a job." Some people will not care that much, or work as hard. They may just treat going to work as a nine to five job. Their feelings towards it may have cooled down. I have also experienced such highs and lows. [CAN]

Another doctor hoped that "I will never stop at the position where I just do the bare minimum and leave it at that, where I say 'Bye bye. Go out and wait' after having explained about the illness" [CAN].

One doctor who was also quoted under the theme "disillusionment" on how she no longer idealized people or conditions in her profession said:

> When I talk to my colleagues about the discrepancy between expectations and reality, many people are not really "bother[ed]": "This is the way it is. Reality is like this, so just let it be. If you accept it, there's nothing wrong." [...] This doesn't just apply to "medicine," but in "real life" as well: when there's a discrepancy between expectations and reality, then you quickly pick a side, and you'll feel more comfortable. If you stand in the middle, you won't know what to do. [CAN].

This is why she thought:

> People who become doctors have one characteristic, at least in Hong Kong—I can't speak for other places. In Hong Kong, doctors are relatively realistic. This isn't necessarily criticism. They very much "stick to reality." They very quickly reach the stage of 'that's the way it is. Let's be more realistic and do it this way.' [...] Also [...] doctors demand a lot of "stability." [CAN]

Even when she said that her words were not "necessarily criticism," however, she felt conflicted:

> Perhaps not many people "struggle" [with these issues], but if you ask me, I think that sometimes I get very angry. [...] I don't even know whom I'm angry with, but I'm angry nevertheless. But afterwards, there's usually a resolution. If not, then you suffer a lot. The resolution is... there isn't much—one way is to find your own position. [CAN]

Although her discomfort with others remaining at the stage of complacency sparked anger at times, it did not lead to a solution apart from her awareness and wariness of complacency, which she used to guard herself against what she called the attitude of "Whatever; anything goes" that she had at times observed at work:

> There's always a "power struggle" between "demoraliz[ation]" and the strength of your hold on your "value[s]." I've "observe[d]" that some people have never had any "value[s]." That is, they enter the field and just do the job. Such people do not get "demoralize[d]" easily. I have more "value[s]," and become "demoralized" easily. But the problem is when people become "demoralize[d]" to the hilt once they do start to become demoralized. They think "Whatever; anything goes." [CAN]

Such complacency could also be the result of the fear of being blamed when anything went wrong. One doctor commented that for cases that are too complex and too difficult, doctors may think: "Let's not do [anything major]; something bad will happen" [CAN], and be inclined towards "conservative treatment or treatment using medication" [CAN] instead.

> Think about it: the private sector usually handles simple cases. Complex cases are passed back to us. If you don't operate on these, they will die, but if you do, they might still not live. Or if you operate on them and the outcome is not good, they will think that medical mistakes have been made. [...] So more and more doctors these days, they will think, "They [patients] are old now, why don't we not do so much?" [CAN]

This leads to "conservative treatment or treatment using medication." So for cases that are too complex and too difficult, [they think]: "Let's not do [anything major]; something bad will happen" [CAN].

2.3.5 *Strategies to Cope with Work Demands*

Doctors described various coping mechanisms to manage the challenges they faced in their work. These included finding sources of mental and emotional support through alternative ways of thinking and working. They also involved consciously accepting and working with the limitations of time and resources.

2.3.5.1 Preserving Values Beyond Work

Two doctors stressed the importance of having a life outside of work as a source of value and meaning, so that they could take a break from work when they left it, and could draw on it as a source of strength while working. One doctor emphasized that "we need to 'cherish' our 'family,' 'friends,' and 'connections.' 'It's not just [about] the job' [ENG]" [CAN]. He said:

> There must be other things to support you mentally. Only then can you [...] "replenish" your "mental state" and your health. And as you grow older, and you marry and have children, your own health, whether "mental" or "physical," is very important. [...] These things are a "source of strength." Because I have my child at home, I have to be able to let things go, and to learn that after I get off work, there's an "on-call team" and my excellent colleagues [to take over]. So I need to be able to let things go, and not "worry" so much. [CAN]

Another doctor also pointed out that a mental break from work, in various forms, was necessary:

> You have to give yourself time to breathe. So my way is, when I go to work during the day, I concentrate on doing my work well, and try my best to bring fewer things home. When I go home, I leave my time for my [...] children and my spouse. [CAN]

He elaborated:

> You must find your own "work-life balance" so that you can "take a break," whether through "sports," "family," or the "church." The Bible says "Love thy neighbor as thyself" [CAN]. In fact, many people "focus" on the part that says "love thy neighbor" [CAN]. But there's the latter part that says "as thyself" [CAN]. [...] So I think that you must find space for yourself, not push yourself too far, and separate "work" and "life" the best you can. You must find a mode. As to what "format" this takes, this is not important—but you must have some space to allow yourself to take a break. [CAN]

2.3.5.2 Optimizing time

The time demands placed on doctors when working meant that interviewees had to plan their time very carefully, rushing through cases when necessary, and arranging any rest time carefully in advance. One doctor said:

> There's never enough time. I think the only thing you can say is that you will do better in a limited amount of time. That is, you do your best. Perhaps you need to plan your time in even more detail and more carefully. For instance, perhaps I need to see 15 to 20 cases in one [specialist] "session." I may do some "planning": in the first 45 minutes, I will rush, and then I will give myself a 10-minute break. I have to "repair" myself "physically" so that I can do my best in the next "round." So I need to "plan" my work even more carefully and even better so that I can handle things better at all times. [CAN]

Another doctor said:

> Perhaps I know that in the coming two weeks I will be very busy, and my own state is such that I haven't rested enough. Maybe I have some patients in my outpatient clinic who are relatively stable. Normally when my state is better, I would try to understand their situation better. But [when I'm not in a good state] I would not necessarily give them so much time, but instead concentrate my energy on some cases that have had problems come up or require some treatment. I can only make adjustments in this regard.

She also pointed out that "when I notice my own state, I try to arrange things better to allow myself to rest a bit. I do some things that are not as urgent later [...]. In terms of time management, leaving myself some space to rest is in fact helpful" [CAN]. Such rest time could:

> be very simple: perhaps it's simply—when I have the time, when I have a 15-minute break—to go and take a walk. In those 15 minutes, I don't think about anything. [...] Before, when I didn't pay attention to my own state, I wouldn't think that 15 minutes made any difference. Perhaps I would do other things. When I pay attention to my own state, and I try different methods, it's a bit better. [CAN]

Such time management strategies became part of doctors' unofficial training. One doctor said:

> Maybe your supervisor can help reduce your "workload" a bit, but when you have many things to do, your own "time management" has to be good. You need to allocate the right time for each thing, and finish that within the allotted time before the second thing. I think that this is what we have become trained in over so many years, that is, you need to be both fast and careful. [CAN]

This means that workload demand might gradually improve even with higher seniority, primarily due to time management strategies improving. Another doctor said:

> Why did I want to become a doctor when I was little? Because when watching TV dramas, I thought it would be very "chill," that you'd be able to go have drinks with "friend[s]" after work. But returning "back to reality," I discovered that this was impossible. When I started off, perhaps because my pace was especially slow [as] a "beginner," in the first few months, "basically" I would get off work only at 9 or 10 pm. At that time, I indeed felt it was tough. But of course, with "experience," the situation slowly improved. "Eventually" "work-life balance" became a bit better. [CAN]

He explained his own time management strategies:

> The main thing is still "efficiency," I would say. Because at "public hospitals," the load is really very high, so you need to do things after "group[ing]" them together. I kind of "prioritize" things, for instance if there are some frivolous things, I put them aside and do them last. This is the main [strategy]. In particular, I "feel" that many "young doctors," because they don't know yet how to "prioritize," feel very strained, and this is the source of their stress. I can't say I do it very well, but "at least" I "feel comfortable" right now. [CAN]

2.3.5.3 Optimizing Limited Public Resources

Several doctors described the limitations in resources as something to be worked around, and even as something that could train their resilience and productivity. For instance, one doctor said that since "public hospitals don't have many resources to 'support' you conducting different tests and treatments, you need to use professional knowledge or experience to make up for it" [CAN]. He thought that "although with some things you really do become more slapdash, because you don't have the resources," "because there is a limitation, you need to use your ability" and "your knowledge at this 'limit[ing]' point to look for the greatest 'potential' to help patients," and "to strive for [patients'] best interests and the maximum amount of resources to help them" [CAN]. This, to him, was "the 'meaning' [driving] this generation of doctors" [CAN].

Another doctor said that since "the minimum amount of money" was used, but "the maximum amount of productivity" was expected, "at the end of the day, then, people in Hong Kong work very hard, very fast, very efficiently." A third doctor said:

> There are many people in the public sector, so it has the highest number of rare and difficult-to-treat diseases. Because it's tough in the public sector, because we don't have enough "resources," the more difficulties you have, the more you learn. So no matter if you want to "learn" or gain more "exposure," or to help the most people, in fact the public sector can "serve" such a" purpose." [CAN]

Having limited resources strips the idea of what is necessary down to the very basics, as one doctor explained. He said:

> At public hospitals, I have learned something called the "arrangement" of "resources." Many "investigation[s]" are not strictly necessary. In the "private" sector, the patient can afford to do more very detailed "investigation[s]." But in the public system, because "resources" are "limited," often we choose which ones to do and which ones not to do, or which ones to do first and which ones after. For instance, currently I'm teaching "medical student[s]," and I say that the most important thing about being a doctor is to talk to patients, "tak[ing]" their "history," and doing a "physical exam" so as to arrive at a "diagnosis." A "diagnosis" is made "by the doctor," and not "by investigation." This is something that public hospitals have—I'm not sure whether it's a meaning, but it's a unique place that "train[s]" someone "up," because if I rely on "investigation[s]" to seek a "diagnosis," basically I don't need to see the "patient." If they come in with "back pain," and I tell them do a series of the most advanced "investigation[s]," then I'd be relying on the "report[s]" to tell me what the matter is. But this is not the correct "medical" care. I insist on "history"-taking and a "physical exam." I order things that I think are appropriate, or what is" urgent." [CAN]

Such an environment:

> tests your "history"-taking and "physical exam" skills. That is, what do you actually "suspect" your "patient" of "suffer[ing]" from? What goes first, and what goes after? These things are the most important things in our "training" "all along": "history"-taking, "physical exam[imation], and communication." [CAN]

Another doctor said:

> Down the line, I learned when the appropriate time is to be doing these kinds of interventions or different kinds of life saving procedures or investigations. And even further down the line, I think I have to learn when not to do these investigations or treatments. [...] This is particularly important in Hong Kong, with the limited resources we have, and just with the load.

2.3.5.4 Focusing on Long-Term Goals

Because working conditions could be so challenging, two doctors gave the advice to focus not on the difficulties of the here-and-now, but on one's entire career trajectory. One doctor said that his advice to medical students would be that:

> Your "vision" needs stretch further. Many people [instead] think, "I'm exhausted right now because I'm on call, and I'm really sleepy." Our "mentor[s]" ask us: "where do you expect yourself to be in five years' time?" So you need to think further ahead. [A colleague told me that] out of 10 or so "new" "medical officer[s] they hired last year, half had already resigned after working for just one year, or less than one year. So to see a bit further ahead is very important, I think. For instance, if you want to be a "kind of regional icon for" a particular "field" after five years, then you'll naturally feel that you can bear things. If every moment you only look at having received many cases while "on call" that night, and on how sleepy you are, then this is definitely "negative feedback." [CAN]

Another doctor said that it was important to "teach [trainees] how to see their 'target,' that is, to see this clearly early on. Sometimes I think that if you like something, you'll continue to 'pursue' it, even if it's tough" [CAN].

2.3.5.5 Grit

Several doctors explained how being merely diligent to deal with the workload was not sufficient, but that extra mental strength and resolve was needed. One doctor called this "grit" [ENG]. He said:

> The work is very busy. I think everyone thinks they're "hardworking," but "diligence" is not enough. You need to have some "grit," because "the work itself" is quite "hard." So when people say "I'm really hardworking, I'm really hardworking," in fact you will still very quickly burn out. [CAN]

Therefore, his advice was: "Don't be 'hardworking for the sake of [being] hardworking.' You have to have some 'grit,' because it's hard work, and long hours" [CAN]. A second doctor said: "I think everyone knows the 'workload' is tough, is heavy. I think your 'mindset' needs to be very firm. If you don't have this willpower, you won't be able to keep going" [CAN].

Two other doctors mentioned the need to just carry on regardless of the conditions. Although this does not at first glance seem very strategic, their conscious approach of acceptance of the situation in the present, and of tackling challenges as they arose, enabled them to continue their work despite the difficulties they faced. One doctor said: "You can only force yourself to endure it. I force myself to. Then you can stay here" [CAN]. Another doctor said when discussing extreme challenges at work: "we just play along as it goes."

2.3.5.6 Increasing Work Efficiency

Apart from planning their time better, as explained with the theme "optimizing time" earlier, doctors also simply, by necessity, used the strategy to go very quickly through the cases they had to handle, trying to do so without compromising patients' safety. One doctor said:

> I think on average, every doctor will see about 20 to 30 patients in a clinic. But for me, my record [is] 50 or 60 patients in the morning. So that's three hours, 60 patients. So that's three minutes per patient. It's not that I want to do this, but then, basically, if you're not fast enough, you will overrun and you don't have time for lunch. [...] Doctors in Hong Kong are trained to be like this since the first day they work at the hospital. [...] So from day one, they are already trained to be fast and efficient. Honestly, the golden rule is to avoid missing very big problems or avoid missing things that would actually kill the patient. And then if the patient is very stable, satisfied, basically, we'll just continue the previous management.

Another doctor jokingly said: "The way to handle it is when more [patients] come, more get taken in" [CAN]. He explained: "I think the simplest way is to do it straight away when you're called upon, and do it faster, and 'train' more people to do things faster" [CAN]. He elaborated:

> For instance, in these past few years, in our "section" that conducts [a specialist procedure], assuming one "section" can "cater" for 4 to 6 [such specialist procedures], then in my "section," I always "overbook" myself by up to 150% to 200%. I just do things faster. [...] There's no choice. No choice. Just do things faster to help patients. [CAN]

A third doctor said:

> My specialty is fortunately a nine to five job, because it's mostly "clinic-based." From nine to five, it's really tough, tougher than "most" other specialties, because even if, for instance, you're a surgeon, you may have "long working hours," in the middle you have a lot of free time while you're waiting around to do "surgery." But in my specialty, the moment you open your clinic, you rush rush rush. But this fits my personality: I like such an "efficient specialty." I think I'd rather do everything I need to do in a very short time, so that I can go home and take care of my children. [CAN]

Drawing on a concrete example, a fourth doctor explained that being efficient also needed to be combined with skilful communication and an empathic perspective, no matter how exhausted he may feel. He said:

> A very simple example would be that there's a typhoon today. We have "clinic[s] in the mornings and afternoons. But because the morning "clinic" has been delayed by the typhoon, a four- or five-hour "clinic" with twenty-odd "patient[s]" has been condensed to perhaps one to two hours in which you have to see twenty-odd "patient[s]." Basically, you will know that you won't be able to see each "patient" for more than five to 10 minutes. So there are definitely "limitation[s]" at outpatient clinics—there must be. But how can we within those five to 10 minutes really "pick up" "patient[s'] chief complaint[s]" and "handle "these? This is a skill. That's the first thing.
>
> The second thing is, how can we in these five to 10 minutes... because my own viewpoint is that in fact the "patient" has waited one to two years to see you, and they will only see you for those five to 10 minutes. In those five to 10 minutes, I know it's tough for many colleagues and they need to rush rush rush, but you should think about things from [the patient's] perspective the best you can, and you should be as calm as you can. Even when you are very impatient and you're exhausted, you should try to understand that they have in fact waited for over a whole year to two years to see you, and all they want is to ask you those few questions. [...] If you can give me one to two hours, I can make them very happy and answer all of their questions, but this isn't possible. But how to answer the questions they're the most "concern[ed]" about in five to 10 minutes, so that they can walk out happily: this is a skill. [CAN]

2.3.5.7 Sustaining Personal Health

Some doctors mentioned the need to keep themselves both physically and mentally healthy as the basis for being able to continue their work in the public sector. One doctor said:

> If you want to be a good doctor, apart from needing to "maintain" good "physical health," your "mental" and "spiritual health" also need to be "strong" enough to "push" yourself to continue. If not, then in fact I've seen many friends either move into the private sector, or go "part-time," or even leave and choose to be a "full-time mom." So I think this is quite important." [CAN]

The doctor whose views on "work-health balance" were quoted under earlier themes said that the "health" in "work-health balance" was in "body, mind, and spirit" [CAN]. She explained:

> These past few years, because the "workload" has been so heavy, I've become a bit more "aware" of "physical need[s]," so now I'm making adjustments towards this direction. I am a person with many interests. I believe the reason why I can "handle" people's "negative emotion[s]" without becoming very depressed myself is because I organize many activities [...]. I know my own needs very well. [...] As doctors, we have to think about many things and take care of many things—of patients, and our own health. If we don't take care of our own health, if I really don't go to the toilet, then I think I would have developed kidney stones a long time ago. [CAN]

2.3.5.8 Mental and Emotional Resilience

If the earlier theme of "grit" revolved around the strength to cope with the heavy workload, the quotations under this theme by two doctors specifically discuss the mental resilience needed to deal with the emotional upheavals that doctors' work necessarily entails. This is because of the inherent risks in medical treatment, as one doctor explained:

> Many people talk about how to have "no risk" in medical treatment. This is impossible. [...] In medical treatment, all procedures carry risk. [...] We can only have "risk minimization," not absolute "risk reduction." This is something we must "get to terms with." We as [specialists] conduct many "procedure[s]," and because there are so many, events occur. [...] When there are complications, we're unhappy, as normal people would be. But how to "handle" these on a mental level, how to adjust—this is something that I've improved a lot in compared with when I first started off. [CAN]

Another doctor recounted her emotions upon hearing a patient's feelings of being dehumanized in his treatment, as previously described under the theme "dehumanization of care":

> The second he finished talking, I already felt that my face was very hot, that I wanted to cry. And then I nodded at him to indicate that I had understood. And then I walked out, because I didn't want him to see me sad, because he was already a very fragile patient. If he knew that his doctor-in-charge was also sad for him, maybe he would feel even worse, so I decided to leave the ward. [...] You can say that I "train" myself to be stronger the best I can, because what we "handle," these people's "suffering"... We cannot even go to the toilet during work—even going to the toilet makes me feel "guilty." And then I need to take care of these people. [CAN]

Since "other people's negative emotions are what we as doctors encounter on a daily basis," she had "become better and better at managing these" over time, and was "still learning this 'resilience'" [CAN]. One way of building up this resilience was to widen her perspective:

> In my daily life, if I encounter any difficult situations, I "actively ""see[k] help." This may not be "seek[ing] help" of a person. Perhaps I "seek help" from "YouTube." When I have a problem that is bothering me, I can type it into "YouTube," and will be able to see many different "perspective[s]." Or I read some books, and I find some different "perspectives." [CAN]

2.3.5.9 Accepting the Gap Between Ideals and Reality

Previously, under the theme "disillusionment," we discussed instances when doctors felt that their actual work fell short of the meanings and ideals they endowed their profession with. Under this present theme, we include quotations that describe doctors' strategy of acceptance of this gap in order to carry on with their work. This acceptance, as the quotations below show, was something that doctors had carefully considered for themselves instead of assuming that it should apply. As one interviewee succinctly put it, sometimes "you have to accept the unwanted in life" [CAN].

One doctor explained how, because of her patient load, the times that she was able to be her ideal type of doctor were fleeting:

> We need to be consider clinical management of the patient, and then we need to consider their feelings, and then we need to listen—sometimes when you don't allow patients to speak, they might think that they're not being understood. Since we only have the opportunity of a very short consultation time, sometimes we do need to cut it short. I can't say that I can touch each case's heart and treat their souls—this is not possible. Within the setting of public hospitals, it is only under certain circumstances—perhaps very critical moments when we have the time—that I can enact the style of the ideal doctor in my mind. [CAN]

She knew conditions were not perfect, and that they did not allow her to be "the ideal doctor" she wanted to be. Yet she did not let this stop her from continuing to treat patients to the best of her abilities and circumstance.

Another doctor also said: "All we can do is do our best. I can't say that we do things really well, but no matter what, there's a 'standard'" [CAN]. Therefore, he advised that "you need to adjust your own 'expectation[s].' [...] If not, then you'll always think something is insufficient" [CAN]. For example, he explained how it could be a struggle to face the death of familiar patients:

> When you have follow-up appointments with [patients], you see them all the time. You will have treated some of them for many years. But in the end, because their condition worsens, they leave. Sometimes you will feel that it's as if you have lost a friend. [...] At least you did what you could do. In the end, the family sometimes also understand. But you will think back, at some point, and you will think that someone very familiar has left. You'll find it hard to let go. [CAN]

However, instead of deadening his emotions, an acceptance of the limits of what he could do helped him continue his work:

> I wouldn't say that we are numb, because if we're too numb then we can't do what we have to do now. For some things, if we can objectively help, then we help, but sometimes when we can't do it, we need to tell them that there are some things that I really cannot do, that everyone has done everything they can. [CAN]

A third doctor elaborated on her reasoning process in embracing acceptance when reality fell short of ideals:

> For instance, [...] we always learned that communication with patients needs time, care, and detail. In reality, time does not allow this: we have too little time to give each patient. This is something we face every day, "day in day out," up to this day. If I continue to work for 30 more years, it will still be a problem. So if you have to do this, you only have two choices. One is, you continue at the speed that you require. For instance, if others can only give you seven minutes, you give [the patient] 15 minutes. Then your patients need to wait double the time, and you will get off work late, and won't be able to go for lunch. Or else you give up, and you won't say that much to the patient, and everyone just says one or two sentences and lets [the patient] go. I believe this is what the majority of doctors are doing.
>
> So in the end you have to be selective. That is, if I feel there is the need, I use my own method. I don't care how long you need to wait, or how much time I need. At the very least, for that one instance that I think is a "case in need," I go back to "serv[ing]" my own "principle." But for the rest, I do my best to fit them into the system. There has to be some give-and-take. If not, it is difficult to continue to work.
>
> So that's how I handle the gap [between ideals and reality]. And I think it has to do with your "personal growth." If you're more "matur[e]," you will "somehow" accept the discrepancy between reality and expectations relatively more easily, not just in work, but in everything.

> You will feel it's "okay," so you won't be as disappointed. You must treat it as a "new understanding of reality." [CAN]

Acceptance could come from knowing that one had done the best one could to help patients, even when the outcome was not what one would have wished for, as a fourth doctor described. He said:

> I've always thought that I have to be very careful, because many things can go wrong. […] If, because you're not careful, something [bad] happens, then no matter what, you won't get over it. If you've really tried your best, and you were very careful and "minimize[d]" [every risk], and in the end something happens, then really there's nothing to be done, but of course you will be a bit unhappy. You will also need to learn how to explain what happened to patients and their family. [CAN]

He explained that it was important to know when to accept that the most ideal scenario, according to doctors' own view, could not be attained due to real-world conditions and human factors:

> I think we need a certain flexibility here. If not, you'll become very worked up. [Say that] you know that an angioplasty procedure is the best for a patient, but they absolutely refuse to have it done. Then in fact, you can't force them, so you have to just let it be. You don't need to get too "worked up about it." "At the end of the day," it's their own decision. "That's why" we're not robots. That is, it's not as if we can input everything and the best "option A" will appear. That's not the case. […] [Patients'] own worldviews and all kinds of other things will add up to their own decision. "At the end of the day," we have to "respect" their "choice." "But" what we need to do is to explain things in a detailed way, to the best of our ability, in the hope that they can "make" that best choice. [CAN]

2.3.5.10 Harnessing Teamwork

Two doctors discussed teamwork as way to mitigate their individual workload. One doctor said:

> "Workload" definitely won't diminish, that is, the size of the cake is definitely very big. The question is, do you eat it all yourself, or can you give some to people to help you handle it? Or you handle it all yourself, but others can at least help you with the layer that sticks out the most. [CAN]

Another doctor said:

> You need to learn that one person cannot do the whole thing, that there's a team as "support," that your colleagues can help. I think I have learned that no matter how much "passion" you have, one person cannot do everything. You really need to have a team, to have people doing things with you. Within this "system," you can't do things by yourself. [CAN]

2.3.5.11 Turning Negatives into Positives

Several doctors were able to see the positive in a wide range of negative aspects in their work. This was an important mental strategy that allowed them to find additional meaning and value in their work and retain the drive to continue their work despite the hardships that could arise.

Two doctors discussed how even though most patient feedback they received may be in the form of complaints, it was still important to focus on the few cases of patients expressing gratitude and praise for their work. One doctor said:

> Although they [patients] won't necessarily thank you, I feel happy inside. Most patients at public hospitals won't thank you now. It's very different: before when I graduated during SARS, many patients would thank you. But thinking further about this, in fact I don't need to have people thanking me. [CAN]

He knew that "no matter how well you do, there will be people who will complain about you. But I look at it with equanimity. As long as I'm able to help them, even if they don't know, or they don't thank me..." [CAN]. Such "equanimity" helped him focus on being "able to help them" no matter whether patients ended up happy with him or not. Another doctor said:

> It's important to find some "positive feedback" to "maintain" your "morale." [...] Seeing so many "case[s]" may be very tough, but thinking of it the other way around, perhaps one or two of those cases will really thank you, even if 20 to 30 cases ignore you. [...] Even when they lodge complaints, only remember the good cases. Quickly wipe away the unhappy cases. [CAN]

A third doctor was similarly able to turn away from negative emotions and find sources of happiness in other places. She said:

> The fluctuations in my emotions can be very big. But when I feel emotionally low, I don't let myself continuously stay in a very low place. Perhaps at this moment, when I think back about something, I feel unhappy, but very soon, I will... For instance, right now [at the time of the interview] I'm at home, and there are other things that can make me happy again. [CAN].

Additionally, she was able to channel the negative emotions she felt into a driving force for her work: "I have discovered that these 'negative emotion[s]' are 'motivational.' I won't want to leave [the public sector] because of these 'moments' that make me want to cry" [CAN]. She thought that her ability to channel these negative emotions without being permanently affected by them was, or had become, natural to her: "I have discovered that [...] my 'emotional capacity' allows me to be like this, without being depressed in any way" [CAN]. She had also learned this approach from observing her patients' response to adversity:

> Sometimes I also learn from patients. Some patients won't stay down because of their diagnosis [of a serious disease]. [...] [They] are very different. There was a patient I remember very well, whom I prescribed 17 medications for, and she said: "It doesn't matter. To treat my illness, I need to take these." And then another patient, I think I prescribed seven for her, and she said: "Wow, there are so many medications to take. Doctor, I don't want to take them. If I have to continue like this, I'm not going to be able to cope." That patient was very "depressed." So one patient had to take 17 medications, and didn't think anything of it. Another patient had to take 7 medications, and felt very "depressed." You can see how their personalities hugely affect their "perspective[s]" towards their disease. I think in these past 10 years or so, I sometimes learned from these "living example[s]." She just needed

to shift her "perspective," and as a result she was able to think that she could live with her disease. And from her "lifestyle," you would not have been able to tell that she was ill. So to some extent I learn from such people. When you encounter a difficult situation, you don't just have one way to... or it doesn't just have one outcome. [CAN]

2.4 Final Remarks

The list of themes presented in this chapter offer a foundation for reflecting on and discussing the work of public hospital doctors in Hong Kong. It is open-ended rather than exhaustive or definitive. The scope of the list, for instance, has been influenced by the greater space made available for its expression due to this being a book-length study, so that we were able to present themes with much finer distinctions between them. As another example of a factor that would have influenced the themes, a greater number of interviewees, from an even wider variety of backgrounds, would again have shaped the list.

Perhaps most importantly, the list has primarily served as an organizational tool to provide structure to the interview narratives in this study, whereas the interview quotations themselves—in which doctors described the joys and the struggles of their work—are ultimately the most edifying and inspiring. These have shown us the multitude of ways in which doctors viewed and expressed their work, and the spectrum of reflections, experiences, and moments that shaped their journey.

The next and final chapter will explore some of the larger issues that emerge from the interview data, and their implications for doctors' work in the Hong Kong public hospital.

References

Labov, W., & Waletzky, W. (1967). Narrative analysis: Oral versions of personal experience. In J. Helms (Ed.), *Essays on the verbal and visual Arts* (pp. 12–44). University of Washington Press.

Wengraf, T. (2001). *Qualitative research interviewing: Biographic narrative and semi-structured methods*. Sage.

Chapter 3
Concluding Reflections

Abstract This chapter critically re-evaluates a selection of the themes that emphasized the interpretive dimension of doctors' experience, and explores their relevance for doctors' work in the Hong Kong public hospital. The chapter will discuss four strands that relate several themes together: work as a public good, work as part of communities, doctors' negotiations of the ideal of the "good" doctor, and an ethics of care predicated on empathy and emotion. The selection of these four strands was based on their alignment with the study's approach and objectives of focusing on subjective meaning-creation in doctors' public hospital work.

Keywords The public hospital sector in Hong Kong · Narrative medicine · Doctors' work as a public good · Doctors' work as part of communities · The ideal of the good doctor · Ethics of care in the medical profession · Empathy and emotion in the medical profession · Human values in the medical profession · Meanings and values in the medical profession · Hong Kong public hospital doctors' work narratives · Interpreting medical practice through narrative · Quality of life and work for medical doctors · The lived experience of medical practice · Reflexivity in medical practice · Narrative research in the health sciences

The previous chapter detailed the themes that emerged from the interview narratives. Some of these, particularly those grouped under "work problems in public hospitals," would not have come as a surprise to readers. In response to these persistent and well-known challenges, various expert suggestions have been proposed throughout the years. A recent policy forum held in July 2023 on "building a sustainable healthcare system for Hong Kong" once again highlighted the familiar issues facing the public healthcare sector faces. Some of the recommendations made by speakers and scholars at the forum could help alleviate the severity of the work-related problems raised by interviewees in this study. For example, Peter P. Yuen's speech (2024), in line with the government's push to "develop a community-based primary healthcare system," suggested the importance of shifting resources and patients towards primary, community-based, and ambulatory care instead of retaining the current model where public hospitals are allocated the bulk of public funding, but where

E. T. Y. Chan and S. Wong, *Doctors' Work in the Public Hospital Sector in Hong Kong*, Quality of Life in Asia 22, https://doi.org/10.1007/978-981-96-6695-9_3

around half of admitted patients could in fact be managed outside them (p. 112). As another example, David T. Y. Lam's speech (2024) summarized a survey he had conducted in 2022 on why staff were leaving the HA, which found that respondents liked "the ability to manage critical illnesses and emergencies, the opportunity to receive training, and a chance to take care of the underprivileged," but disliked the "heavy workload in the Hospital Authority," and its "very bad governance" (pp. 18–19). The private sector was, in contrast, appealing because of "work-life balance," and "A higher income" (p. 19). Despite the familiarity of these challenges, the value in hearing interviewees recount some of these problems in this study, as mentioned in the Introduction, lies less in pushing towards specific solutions—especially since some proposed solutions already exist and merely await implementation—and more in reading about doctors' own experiences, in their own words (even if in translation), and using their own examples and views.

Many other themes that focused more on the individual meanings and values that their public hospital work held for doctors, and their struggles and strategies to retain and sustain these even as they faced adversity in their work, were more unique findings. For these, doctors' rich, first-person descriptions provided illuminating insights into the personal and professional conflicts they faced. Within and across these themes, the previous chapter revealed the major tensions between the personal meanings and ideals that doctors endowed their hospital work with, and the chaotic reality of doctors' work.

The aim of this final chapter is not to rehearse these findings, which are largely self-explanatory. Instead, this chapter will critically re-evaluate a selection of the themes in relation with each other to arrive at a deeper understanding of doctors' negotiations with their work. We propose four strands for discussion in this chapter. The first and second strands that combine multiple themes are the conception of doctors' work as a public good and as an integral part of communities both of which give important meaning to doctors' work in the public sector in Hong Kong. The third strand is doctors' movement between personal meanings, values, and ideals, and the realities of their work. This can be summarized as a process of negotiation, where doctors moved between the positions of aspiration to ideals and values on the one hand, and of compromise in the face of less-than-ideal work conditions on the other. The final strand focuses on the value of empathy and emotions, which hinges in the narratives on seeing patients as more than two-dimensional clinical cases, whether during the consultation itself, or as part of doctors' own reflection on the humanity of patients outside of the clinical encounter. Altogether, these strands distil some of the meanings and values of public hospital work in Hong Kong for the doctors interviewed, and the ways in which they continued to hold onto and shape these throughout their careers.

3.1 Work as a Public Good

As the Introduction explained, public hospitals in Hong Kong provide around 90% of in-patient care, yet the total number of doctors in Hong Kong is shared almost equally by the public and private healthcare sectors, creating a disproportionate patient load. On the one hand, the workload this entails could disincentivize doctors from staying in public hospitals. On the other hand, one insight gained from the narratives in this study is interviewees' keen awareness of how much they were needed by the huge number of patients in the public system. This strong motivator for them to stay in the public system shaped themes such as "feeling indispensable" and "patients from all walks of life," to the extent that we used the term "interpellation" to refer to doctors' sense of being essential to the public hospital system, which became a part of their work identity. What was therefore crucial to interviewees was the word "public" in their work identity as public hospital doctors, where their work comprised a public good.

Other themes such as "non-materialist thinking," "work as a higher calling," "duty to patients and society," and "instigating social change" highlight additional interactions between the notions of "public" and "doctor" in the identity of the public hospital doctor. The idea of medicine as a public good is characterized by equitable access for everyone, so that no one can be excluded from using it. Where doctors discussed their sense of duty and obligation, and the meanings they derived from their work, as escaping the professional bounds of their work, their descriptions moved towards the idea of their work as a civic and social rather than a purely professional duty. These findings on the importance doctors placed on their work as a public good correspond to those in some existing research on doctors' work identity. One particularly relevant study of doctors working at large hospitals in South Korea has shown that "while medical doctors are likely to be satisfied with their jobs when they work at either purpose-driven or profit-driven hospitals, only purpose-driven hospitals give doctors a sense of meaningfulness" (Chang et al., 2022, p. 641). The study found "a concealed mechanism of meaningfulness," where "meaningfulness" is "a part of public service motivation concept, which prescribes how people thrive in their lives by serving the benefits of others," instead of being driven solely by profit (Chang et al., 2022, p. 641). The authors discovered that this sense of meaningfulness "still holds when workloads (e.g., work hours or number of patients under one's care) are controlled for," "impl[ying] that meaningfulness is central to their career identity and may not be easily compromised by other external motivating schemes or forces" (Chang et al., 2022, p. 641). As we have seen, interviewees in this book expressed this sense of meaning in their role as agents of public good in their work in different ways. One example is the sense of dedication and pride we have observed in an interviewee we quoted, who said: "I'm able to say these cool words all the time: 'This is a public hospital. I only treat and manage this disease. Although we have limited resources, we will use the best and the most 'proper' ways to treat you. Do not talk to me about money—this is irrelevant'" [CAN]. Another example is the strong sense of responsibility to serve the greater good that we have seen in a different interviewee we quoted, who thought that "If God gave you the ability to be a doctor, you have to make good use of this ability to help people in need, 'rather than' moving to the private sector to earn big money" [CAN].

The public system also enabled doctors' work to serve as a public good in an additional way, despite the headwinds being discussed by interviewees: there was the space for doctors to go for further training in response not only to individual interest, but also the public system's needs, and to have the resources and space to conduct research that contributed to medical science, with a particular focus on the applicability in Hong Kong. In themes such as "further training and enhanced learning" and "research work," interviewees contrasted the availability of these to the relative lack of these in the private sector. This applied on a more subjective dimension as well: doctors' own intellectual curiosity could find more fulfilment in service of the public good, and find greater meaningful and productive outlet.

For the doctors we interviewed, these, together with other factors, had so far provided sufficient incentive to stay. However, interviewees also discussed how their ideal of public service was being eroded by some of the systemic work conditions they faced, such as their very heavy patient load, and the rules and regulations in place that saw the treatment of patients primarily in terms of numbers and figures. These were expressed in themes such as "high workload," "dehumanization of care," "departure from patient-centric care," and "bureaucratic barriers." For instance, one interviewee we quoted whose passion for her public hospital work was very obvious for the entire duration of an interview that lasted almost two hours said that even she went through a period before when she "became a bit lost as I worked," when her workload was so heavy that she "felt that it was eroding my willpower" and "that passion" [CAN]. Another doctor, as we saw, lamented the HA's emphasis on "making the numbers look better," for instance on "how many days it takes to discharge people" [CAN], instead of taking an approach that centered on patients' needs. Although this approach to the management of patient load is an important part of the allocation of resources in public health, the patient volumes that many public hospital doctors have to manage each day is premised on a static data-centric approach to the achievement of outcomes—as one doctor quoted put it, the assumption that if "previously 10 patients could be seen in one session," then the rhetorical question that should follow would be: "so why can't you see 10 patients now?" [CAN]. Such a question does not yet allow for a consideration of a more patient-centric approach, which would allocate fewer patients to doctors so that there could be more time for good communication between doctor and patient, and the establishment of good doctor-patient rapport.

In the arena of public health, such phenomena are not entirely unique to Hong Kong. The situation where "Clinicians increasingly feel diminished and disempowered" as they are "caught in the maw of bureaucratic documentation and burdensome regulation, estranged from the call to care and the intimacy of the doctor-patient relationship" has been documented in both academic studies and alternative narrative sources, such as "memoirs by physicians" that "recount experiences of profound bewilderment, humiliation, fatigue, brutality, and a loss of empathy and idealism" (Irvine & Spencer, 2017, p. 68). However, the accessibility of Hong Kong's public hospital service, the extent of its use, and the overallocation of public health patients to this system rather than to primary or community-based care (Yuen, 2024, pp. 111–112)[1] underscore the extremes of the Hong Kong public hospital sector that interviewees highlighted. The "public" aspect of public hospitals is then both a source of pride, and a source of worry, as interviewees pointed out. They create troubling individual statistics for public hospital doctors that lurk in the background: of, on average, "need[ing] to see 20 to 30 patients" "in one shift of three hours," which amounts to "five minutes per patient" [CAN], although, as we have read, one doctor's personal record was "50 or 60 patients" in "three hours."

Projections of big public healthcare expenditure increases as Hong Kong's population continues to age may push the concerns discussed above to the side, in preference of debates that seem enormously pressing, such as on the affordability of public healthcare expenditure in future, and on how to restructure public health service so that a better developed primary healthcare system can take some of the pressure off public hospitals and increase its overall "allocative efficiency" (Yuen, 2024, p. 112). However, although prioritizing must inevitably take place, the above issues raised in the interviews also deserve some consideration in conjunction with the other crucial concerns relating to the sustainability of the public healthcare sector in Hong Kong. It is clear from the interviews that many doctors felt a sense of pride in being indispensable members of a public hospital system that still managed to deliver good outcomes for an enormous number of patients without regard for patients' financial status or personal material interests. The *public* aspect of their work created a sense of calling that kept interviewees in it, despite the work conditions they described. Such dedication to their work as a public good should be acknowledged, strengthened, and consolidated by addressing the problems raised in this strand, and not continuously "erod[ed]," as one interviewee put it, by conditions detrimental to both doctor and patient.

3.2 Work as Part of Communities

In his book *Community, Solidarity and Belonging*, Andrew Mason (2000) uses the strictly professional doctor-patient relationship as an example of a "non-communal relationship," predicated on doctors' "professional roles" (p. 29). He contrasts this with communal relationships, and proposes the notion of "solidarity"—which he sees as "mutual concern"—as underpinning the idea of community (p. 27). He writes that this mutual concern "minimally [...] means that members must give each other's interest some *non-instrumental* [emphasis added] weight" (p. 27). Without excessively overlayering this discussion with theoretical debates on the notion of "community," since this would exceed the scope of this study, this section builds on this idea of "community" that is underpinned by the idea of "solidarity" to reconsider

[1] For a discussion of the background to, and recommendations for, developing a "community-based primary healthcare system" to relieve the pressure on public hospital service in Hong Kong, see Health Bureau (2023).

some of the themes from the last chapter. Although we use Mason's definition, in our discussion of the strand of doctors' work as part of communities in this section, we in fact move away from Mason's use of doctors' work roles as an example merely of "professional roles" and therefore of a "non-communal relationship" (p. 27). Indeed, in the interviews in this study, it was difficult to disentangle doctors' sense of pure professional duty to patients, and their sense of responsibility to the wider community and society underpinned by a sense of solidarity. Interviewees' sense that they were located in, and played an integral role in, communities that they were a part of and had a stake in could be observed in themes such as "duty to patients and society," "patients from all walks of life," "teaching the next generation of doctors," and "empowering teamwork." Such a sense of community derived from both the setting of Hong Kong and their workplace community, where colleagues, mentors, mentees, and students further ensconced doctors in a meaningful web of relations.

The strand in this section on doctors' work as part of communities can be seen as an extension of the idea of "work as a public good" just discussed, but with a somewhat different focus. In emphasizing the "reciprocal community of relationships" (Green-Thompson et al., 2017, p. 269) between members, where interviewees felt themselves to be part of their community because of a shared background and story, this strand contains a more storied dimension than the previous strand. For instance, an interviewee we quoted thought that she owed a duty of care to the Hong Kong community and society that her life had been embedded in since birth, which she saw as having raised and nurtured her:

> I come from a very poor family. But I applied for whatever subsidy I could. I remember we had very little money to spend towards my studies. [...] So basically, my entire learning and study journey, and strictly speaking the "degree" I obtained, was paid for by "taxpayers." [...] The taxpayers from when I was little are now all "elderly"—perhaps they're all retired. Those retired people very often cannot afford to go "private," because they don't have money. So they end up in the public system as part of the "aging population." So sometimes, when I see that "population," I think: these people paid for my education when I was young, paid for my tuition fees perhaps. [CAN]

The interviewee had developed a reciprocal relationship of accountability and responsibility with members of the community, as part of a self-imposed social compact with them, so that it was as if they were her family whom she needed to take care of in their old age. Serving them through work was an extension of her upbringing and growth in the Hong Kong community and society.

An additional type of community we can identify in the data is the workplace community that doctors were part of in public hospitals. This, as the narratives made clear, comprised not only strictly occupational connections, but was also a community of learning, growth, and emotional support, where the sense of having a social and moral—and not just professional—duty to support colleagues and pass on the torch to the next generation of doctors was very strong. This community was often discussed as a distinct advantage of the public system. For instance, as we have seen, doctors frequently mentioned that they would not be able to have the same opportunities to collaborate so closely with other doctors, and train the next generation of doctors, in the private sector. Interviewees also often highlighted how teamwork, a crucial component of public hospital work that is not a prominent feature of private sector work, was invaluable beyond the acquisition of technical knowledge, as exemplified in the interview quotations under the theme of "empowering teamwork." And they frequently mentioned having benefited from mentorship themselves while working towards various professional milestones. The idea of the workplace as a community thus contained the story of past nurturing engendering a continuing duty and responsibility, as did the earlier idea of being part of a Hong Kong community. This is expressed in an interview quotation we have seen:

> Many people leave after they've finished "train[ing]." It is really disappointing to us. From the perspective of a "team," of course if you lose a colleague, the dullest way of expressing this is that you lose one pair of hands: "do you want to work us to death?" [...] But in fact I think there's something else that leads to me feeling very disappointed. [...] I'm very grateful I have a group of very good "senior[s]" who gave us a lot of care and knowledge and time to nurture you, to teach you. You really "work as a team," and you really work and strive hard together. [...] But why when everyone spent so much effort to nurture you, do you just leave with a swish? [...] It is without doubt very "stressful" and very exhausting [work], but it's something "meaningful." [CAN]

The idea of reciprocal responsibility expressed here is very similar to that expressed in the interview quotation earlier. The "mutual concern" that is solidarity, whereby members of a community "give each other's interest some *non-instrumental* [emphasis added] weight" (Mason, 2000, p. 27) is based not on a purely professional or externally imposed contractual obligation, but on having weaved and contributed to a shared story of formative growth that does not end merely when formal training ends, but should extend beyond this point.

The two interview passages re-quoted above also show how being ensconced in communities can help doctors tell the narratives about themselves that establish their identity and values. It is through calibrating oneself within these communal relations that it becomes possible to position one's work in stronger relation to the wider community, creating a moral story and language of duty, responsibility, and reciprocity. From a strictly professional and administrative perspective, it may seem unsuitable to use such morally inflected language to discuss doctors' work in public hospitals in Hong Kong. However, there is good reason for interviewees to draw on such ways of expression when employing the narrative mode to explain their work, since the consideration of the idea of community is intrinsically related to such moral ideas. In Hong Kong, strengthening such ways of seeing and discussing doctors' work, without forceful imposition of such ideals on doctors—of attempting to hold them morally hostage to these ideals, as it were—would help express and validate an important source of meaning to doctors' work.

3.3 Negotiating the Ideal of the "Good" Doctor

In a short essay entitled "A consideration of the qualities of a 'good' doctor with some help from the humanities," Jane Moore (2009) asks the question: if "analysis and surveys, codes of practice, guidelines and protocols cannot define the role of a 'good' doctor then how does the medical profession reconcile the many conflicts presented by the practice of contemporary medicine?" (p. 60). This question summarizes the key issues in the strand under discussion in this section. The interviews, as this section will consider, show the figure of a "good" doctor to be the product of continuous negotiation—for instance between interviewees' ideals of work and its realities, between the meanings and values their work held for them and the headwinds they faced in retaining them, and between the standards they set for their work beyond formal and professional protocol and the exigencies in their work context.

Such personal formulations of a "good" doctor escape definition in clinical textbooks or scholarship, as Moore's question suggests. Yet, as her question also indicates, "a 'good' doctor" is a particularly important evaluation to attempt. The difficulties of defining, shaping oneself into, and remaining a "good" professional practitioner is not a phenomenon unique to the medical profession, since many workers face similar challenges. Indeed, within the very definition of the word "ideal" (or even the word "profession," where one "professes" standards and values in one's work) is embedded the necessary corollary of falling short when faced with real-world conditions, or else a value would not be called an "ideal" but a plan or a method. However, what makes the medical profession more unique is the fact that extreme life-and-death versions of such difficulties play out in it. Doctors "enter the lives of patients in times of great disruption" (Charon, 2011, p. 37), when they are in some of their most vulnerable states, and need to reconcile ideals of the profession "with the emotional messiness of ordinary living and the harried everyday reality of medical practitioners" (Avrahami, 2011, p. 325). These conflicts are in turn exacerbated by the very high patient load, time pressures, and resource constraints that are part and parcel of public hospital work in Hong Kong, which many interviewees discussed. Under such conditions, having clear methods or plans in place for managing patients is imperative, but these can at the same time only go so far in keeping the various meanings, values, and ideals that go into being a "good" doctor intact. Although doctors discussed various specific coping strategies, the idea of constant, processual negotiation can summarize the overall approach that doctors took to make their ideals, meanings, and values of work workable and mouldable within the challenges of their daily work. Such a process of negotiation was not a simple evaluative exercise, where doctors weighed the benefits against the costs of staying in their public hospital work. Rather, it was a constant recalibration, in a variety of directions, of meanings and values in the face of shifting work conditions at different stages of their lives and careers.

Negotiation involved compromise, where, when interviewees were not able to fully achieve what they would ideally like their work to be like, they needed to accept having to lower their own expectations so they could meet the realities of their work and make it practicable. In this sense, the idea of compromise was embedded into many of the themes in the last chapter, but was perhaps most prominently demonstrated in the theme of "accepting the gap between ideals and reality." Here, one doctor was quoted as saying:

> I can't say that I can touch each case's heart and treat their souls—this is not possible. Within the setting of public hospitals, it is only under certain circumstances—perhaps very critical moments when we have the time—that I can enact the style of the ideal doctor in my mind. [CAN]

The doctor's knowledge of her conception of "the ideal doctor" and the desire to fulfil this ideal was contrasted with her awareness of her often falling short of this ideal. Yet she also made it clear that she understood such falling short was inevitable, and that it neither diminished the importance of her work, which she must continue to do, nor of her ideals. Without this strategy of compromise, a fatalism—or "the hazard of disillusionment in medicine itself, when ideals and reality come into conflict" (Spiegel & Spencer, 2017b, pp. 39–40)—could set in that could erode the integrity of medical ideals to the extent where doctors "treat going to work as a nine to five job" [CAN], as one interviewee described under the theme "the risks of complacency."

Negotiation also involved aspiration towards higher ideals, meanings, and values, which moves in the opposite direction of compromise. If the realities of their work were less than ideal, then constantly looking towards work ideals, standards, and values also helped interviewees keep sight of these, even when doctors knew that in reality they could not be fully enacted, or at least not all or most of the time. For instance, under the theme of "keeping one's initial idealism close," doctors described constantly reminding themselves of the ideals they had started their studies or careers with, so that even in their most hectic or troubled moments, their work conditions did not fully overwhelm and dissipate the self-authored meaning of their work. They accommodated the chaos of practical work conditions, but resisted complete loss of idealism.

Work ideals were also not always static, and had to respond to and be redefined in the face of real-life work conditions and the accumulation of practical experience and coping strategies. For instance, one doctor was quoted as discussing how he had changed from thinking of his work as putting him "in a very esteemed position" at the beginning of his career to gradually understanding and embracing the value of humility in his work:

> The younger you are, the more you think that being a doctor or being in a "medical" profession is something very esteemed, very "above," very "superior." But in fact when you really start working, you will discover that you must chat with "patient[s]" in a very down-to-earth way to understand them, and only then can you really help them. [CAN].

However, the very process of thinking about their ideals and values prevented interviewed doctors from giving fully in to the brutal pragmatism that work conditions could demand. Although they were not able to be their version of an ideal doctor at all times or to all patients, knowing that they aspired to ideals was enough to keep the personal meanings they endowed their work with going, even when these needed to take a backseat to the chaos of real-life working conditions.

Retaining ideals through the dual movements of compromise and aspiration as part of doctors' constant negotiation can serve as a bulwark against depersonalization and against work turning impersonal due to harsh challenges and conditions, which comes with a high risk for burnout (Busireddy et al., 2017; See et al., 2018; Siu et al., 2012; West et al., 2018). Yet having observed the importance of this process of negotiation, we also note that ideals can chastise and constantly lead to feelings of inadequacy that may undermine, rather than promote, doctors' competent work.[2] If ideals are so much embraced and become so much part of one's personal narrative that the inability to attain them is a source of constant guilt and even shame, this can become self-destructive and debilitating. And we can also surmise what might happen if the space for doctors to negotiate with their ideals is completely crowded out—if they were so busy that they could not even hope to partially attain some of the ideals they held dear.

Negotiation as *movement*—as part of "Finding and maintaining a functional critical stance" (Spiegel & Spencer, 2017a, p. 25)—is therefore crucial, instead of standing still at any one point, whether this be the point of having no ideals, or fixating on them to the extent of seeing oneself as a failure when one finds it impossible to live up to them. If there were to be a narrative syntax for such negotiation, it would take the following form: "*Despite how* this is the reality, I can *still* take this action, or think in this way." This introduces a dynamic of personalization and humanization of work. The goal is neither to attain perfection, nor to lose the encouragement and chastisement of ideals.

The idea of doctors' work as negotiation that can be observed from the interview data pushes back against the figure of the doctor as "a collection of competencies produced by medical education in a 'manufacturing model' of medical training" (p. 249), as Bennett et al. (2017) have discussed. Such a "discourse of competence" "contribut[es] to the assumption of a standardised 'good doctor' produced through training" (p. 249). Yet becoming a doctor is not "a uniform set of values, attitudes and behaviours" that culminates in "a 'completed' process of professional identity formation," and "[t]his narrowing of focus does not acknowledge the possibility of diverse trajectories and variations between doctors in how they interpret and develop their professional identities" (p. 249). Although there are of course rigorous common standards, "the standardisation discourse does not recognise that medical students and doctors actively construct diverse identities under the broad umbrella of the 'good doctor'" (p. 249). If "Professional culture has little space for personal becoming" (Spiegel & Spencer, 2017b, p. 40), viewing medical work not only in terms of outcomes and competencies, of specialist training and exams passed, but also as a journey that doctors constantly negotiate for themselves, and aspects of which narrative form might be better placed to describe, lies at the core of the strand of negotiation in this section, and indeed of the present study's approach. In this way, the emphasis is on doctors writing their own identity of a "good doctor," one that is

---

[2] This is what Spiegel and Spencer (2017a) describe as "the negative impact of the narrative of 'The Heroic Doctor,' a staple of medical and popular culture" (p. 25).

not static but shifts over time in response to agency, circumstance, requirements, and needs.

The danger here, however, is also of taking the idea of the need for negotiation to the extreme, no matter the extent, and without regard for doctors' physical and mental wellbeing. Asking doctors to be fully flexible to accommodate real conditions and get the work done, while still embracing the meanings and ideals of their work, may not seem as laudable when reading the following interviewee's words, quoted previously:

> Within, above, and below [my rank], there is no one, so I'm the representative of this span of 10 years' [experience]. So people [ranking] above me ask me to do things to help them, and colleagues [ranking] below me also ask me. I'm doing things that are the most front-line, but I also do logistical things. All work duties "overlap" and are draped over my shoulders. I don't even know what my upcoming "duties" are, because I'm almost like a "relieving" worker, that is, I go wherever there are not enough people. [CAN]

Negotiation as a method to cope with such circumstances should not be imposed as a viable long-term strategy. Indeed, the interviews showed that the need for compromise in the face of dire working conditions could take a grave toll on doctors, and several interviewees indicated that working conditions could be such that the loss of ideals was a danger that was never far away. This specific interviewee, for instance, was also quoted in the previous chapter as talking about "becom[ing] a bit lost as I worked" in the past, because "I just felt that the 'workload' was too 'heavy,' and I felt that it was eroding my willpower. That is, that passion—it was being a bit eroded" [CAN]. There is therefore a balance to be struck between seeing the practical need for negotiating between ideals and reality, and encouraging this negotiation to take place to such an extreme extent that ideals become mere distant memories that are unable to rekindle deeper meanings of work.

3.4 Towards an Ethics of Care: Empathy and Emotions

Our discussion of the strand of "community" touched upon the subjective, storied dimension it contained, where doctors were narratively embedded in the communities that their work had an impact on, and which endowed their work with additional meaning. But this was not the only storied dimension that doctors read in their work. Doctors' responses often focused on how they saw their patients as more than clinical cases to be treated through thinking of them as storied. Whether interviewees talked about the importance of having an empathic approach to patient care in the theme of "balancing empathy and its limits," or engaging in small talk with patients despite their hectic consultation schedule in the theme of "compassionate, effective communication in care," doctors described an ethics of care that was shaped around an empathic consideration of patients as storied human beings. One example quoted in the previous chapter is that of a doctor recounting how he engaged a patient in conversation early on in his career:

> if you just say a bit more, or can "just be more curious" about the "patient," about what they themselves are thinking, or "just" as small talk… At first when I started to chat with him it wasn't for anything specific, but just because I was doing these procedures, and didn't want him them to be bored and staring at what I was doing, and make me even more "stressed." We started talking and […] it was very run-of-the mill the first few times. But subsequently you would hear about how his background was in fact very wretched. […] Very often it's the environment that influences [your situation in life]. […] Sometimes we may only see some "label[s]" that say they're an "IV drug user" and so on. We may "label" a "patient" as a miscreant. In fact, I think "at the end of the day" people are by nature benevolent, but it's just that their "circumstances" or their willpower weakened. So "even if" this is the case, I think "there's always a story behind" every person, and although understanding more may not be necessary "from a clinical point of view," "at least" you can have better "rapport" with the "patient." […] "Every patient" has a "back story behind" them. [CAN]

The patient's story, which started as a way to distract the patient from medical procedures, soon became a new way of understanding him that was redundant from a clinical perspective, but which allowed the interviewee to see the human being behind the purely clinical history and escape the simplistic "label[s]" that failed to define the patient. The series of consultations the interviewee had with the patient demonstrate what Charon (2011) calls "narrative competence," or "the competence that human beings use to absorb, interpret, and respond to stories," which "enables the physician to practice medicine with empathy, reflection, professionalism, and trustworthiness" (p. 1897). Such narrative competence brings together "the personal connections between patient and physician, the meaning of medical practice for the individual physician, physicians' collective profession of their ideals, and medicine's discourse with the society it serves" (p. 1898).

The interviewee's broader recognition that "'Every patient' has a 'back story behind' them" [CAN] also generates an empathic foundation for patients that is not merely an "intellectual" exercise, as according to the model of "detached concern" that is still often used to define clinical empathy (Halpern, 2003, pp. 670–671). Jodi Halpern (2003), in the essay "What is clinical empathy?," explains that this model regards "a special professional empathy as purely cognitive, contrasting it with sympathy" (p. 670). This model's espousal of "*detached* [emphasis added] concern" arises out of the worry that "Sympathetic physicians risk overidentifying with patients" (Halpern, 2003, p. 670). However, Halpern points out, "the function of empathy is not merely to label emotional states, but to recognize what it feels like to experience something" (p. 671). It is an "experiential" and "'perceptual' activity that operates alongside logical inquiry" (p. 673), rather than being itself a process of mere logical inquiry.

Importantly, Halpern argues that such "*engaged* [emphasis added] empathy" does not pose the excessively onerous requirement of "experiencing emotions in parallel with each patient": "empathy does not require that physicians vicariously experience and introspect about patients' emotions" (p. 671). Rather, "Emotional attunement operates by shaping what one imagines about another person's experience. In trying to imagine what the patient is going through, physicians will sometimes find themselves resonating," which is "not a special professional skill, but a part of ordinary communication," and a part of the very act of "imagining" itself (p. 671).

Such "imagining" and "resonance" as "part of ordinary communication" (p. 671), instead of strictly professional communication that seeks to purely gather clinical information, could indeed be observed in the interview quotation we have seen just now, and in the following one by another doctor, quoted in the previous chapter:

> You should think about the "patient['s]" feelings. I think if you try to "shift" your feelings onto patients, you think about what feelings they have first. If the "clinic" is constantly trying to chase you away, maybe you… In fact, the same words but said in a different tone […], or saying a few simple sentences—I think the "impact" is very big on you. That is, your "impact" on others is very big. So I think that I shouldn't be too egocentric, and lay down my ego and try and understand. This is empathy […], where you understand what people's feelings are. I think this is very important. [CAN]

Here, the interviewee did not describe himself as delving deeply into the individual stories of his patients like the first interviewee. However, his imagination of patients' emotions created an emotional "resonance" (Halpern, 2003, p. 671) that changed the way he conceived of his own position as a doctor, and the tone of his consultations. The clinical consultation became an exercise—albeit to an extent that must always be constrained by time and resources, and, as we will soon touch upon, by professional boundaries—in "inventiveness and imaginativeness," instead of "detachment," which is "the adoption of an ideal of objectivity that rests on the assumption that one must remain outside the story of the other" (Irvine & Charon, 2017, p. 116).

The interview data, however, has also revealed one important caveat to consider, with doctors careful to impose limits on such "inventiveness and imaginativeness" (Irvine & Charon, 2017, p. 116) in their empathic response. This observation accords with our discussion of doctors constantly adjusting ideals, meanings, and values in response to real working conditions in the previous section on the strand of negotiation. For instance, the doctors who emphasized the importance of the value of empathy also set workability constraints: although they saw their patients as human beings with their own stories, they also knew the restrictions on their time, energy, and emotional capacity, and understood the necessity of professional boundaries so that they could do their work effectively and appropriately. On the one hand, they applied empathy to ensure that they did not merely see patients as clinical cases to be solved or treated, but as patients whose humanity lay at the basis of their relationship. The second doctor quoted just now constantly reminded himself to "Try to think from the patient's perspective," to imagine how "perhaps they have waited for a long time to be able to see us, or perhaps to them the 'treatment' is a 'life and death treatment,' or it really 'affect[s]' their whole 'family planning' and their entire lives," instead of seeing the patient purely from the perspective of a doctor's workload, as merely "one amongst the 30 'patient[s]' in my 'clinic'" [CAN]. On the other hand, empathy was also just a quick step into the perspective of patients, a brief imagining of patients' stories, serving as an anchor for the clinical encounter rather than comprising it in its entirety. It ensured a moral foundation upon which to ground the clinical encounter, without creating a responsibility to narrativize or story the patient too far.

Appropriately delimiting empathic engagement was therefore crucial to doctors being able to continue to function as doctors. In the last chapter, we quoted an interviewee who described himself as at one point becoming so empathically and sympathetically invested in a patient's story that during a surgery he found himself unable to "put knife to skin" and "br[eaking] down." He could at that moment not perform his work because of the extent of his emotional resonance with the patient. Conversely, the opposite of caring in the form of "compassion fatigue" could also result from insufficiently delimited empathic engagement. Compassion fatigue results in "a disassociation from the people [healthcare workers] are trying to help, and diminished joy in their work that can be outwardly exhibited as a lack of empathy, emotional distancing, defensiveness or even displays of anger" (Fisher et al., 2022, p. 641). A further negative consequence that has been mentioned before may be burnout, which several interviewees discussed, and which, in contrast to compassion fatigue "is more about the long-term effects of being exposed to emotionally draining situations" (Fisher et al., 2022, p. 641).

By putting limitations to empathy in place, "the integrity of the caring person," which "is critical for helping another person," is maintained even as empathy is experienced, expressed, and applied, since "If the person caring for another loses his or her integrity, then that person is unable to make an objective evaluation of what needs to be accomplished to help the other" (Marcum, 2012, p. 111). Caring, in James Marcum's account (2012) in his book *The Virtuous Physician*, requires "appropriate professional boundaries for defining patient-physician dyads so that the relationships are therapeutic for and not harmful to patients," striking a balance "between getting too close to the patient and remaining too distant" (p. 159). As one interviewee in this study, quoted in the previous chapter, also pointed out:

> On the one hand you are very "attached to" your "patient[s]." On the other hand you must "detach" yourself, or else you can't continue to work. So although you are in the relationship of a patient and a doctor, there can't be too many personal emotions. Sometimes it's very difficult to "strike" a "balance." [...] But we have to maintain the right doctor-patient relationship no matter what. That is, you can't "intrude" on their personal lives. On the one hand, you have to understand them. On the other hand, you can't get too involved. [CAN]

This balance ensures that "The virtuous physician does not abuse the power differential or inequity of the therapeutic relationship but rather uses the power entrusted to him or her by both the patient and society to the patient's and society's benefit and welfare" (Marcum, 2012, p. 161).

Additional ways in which Marcum's book discusses the idea of caring—defined in generic terms as "a disposition or an attitude in which a person exhibits a deeply felt concern or empathy" (p. 108)—can help extend our discussion of empathy in the interview data further. Marcum explains the importance of emotions in genuine care in the clinical setting alongside "boundaries," emphasizing that "genuine caring has an emotional component—interest in or concern for humanity—and without that component motivating clinicians to take care of [...] patients, especially patients they may not like, quality healthcare would be next to impossible" (p. 132). Genuine caring is in contrast to mere "care behavior," since without "any emotional connection"—which is the "interest in or concern for humanity" mentioned just now, and "not care qua liking"—there would not be much to "motivate clinicians to be benevolent or to act for the good of their patients" (p. 132). Genuine caring is also in contrast to what Marcum calls "uncaring," which "is a disposition or an attitude of a person who is unable or incapable of feeling any concern or empathy for another person" (p. 132), and which may be the result of "the scientific and technical training in medicine of prospective physicians" that "often brackets from the clinical consultation the patient's illness experience and any emotions associated with it" (p. 2). Such training produces "a medical professional who is emotionally detached from what the patient feels or experiences and who thereby appears uncaring to the patient" (p. 2). While technical knowledge is crucial—especially since "incompetence" also "instantiates uncaring" (p. 125)—caring with an emotional instead of a purely procedural or behavioural basis is also important, a focus that we have seen in interviewees' narratives of work in this study. When we reconsider the story by the interviewee who recounted her patient telling her that he felt that medical personnel in another ward "did not treat him like a human being" while his "tears were falling" [CAN], we see such a demonstration of "genuine caring" as described by Marcum. The interviewee suppressed her own tears while "nodd[ing] at [the patient] to indicate that I had understood" [CAN]. She did not stop her tears to negate her emotions—she described herself as "very much accept[ing] that I am moved by patients' 'suffering' to experience 'negative emotions'" [CAN]. Rather, she refrained from crying herself because she "required my professional image not to be affected, because that would affect the patient: he would question whether this doctor was reliable, and he would be even more scared" [CAN]. Her priority was always the patient: "he was already a very fragile patient. If he knew that his doctor-in-charge was also sad for him, maybe he would feel even worse, so I decided to leave the ward" [CAN]. The interviewee's empathic response stemmed from her sincere emotions, which fundamentally guided her decisions. Instead of "detached concern" (Halpern, 2003, p. 670), she felt genuine, emotion-based concern, yet was able to control her emotions sufficiently in order not to adversely affect the patient's own emotional state. Having felt these emotions keenly, she could also recover quickly and continue her work, explaining that "when I feel emotionally low, I don't let myself continuously stay in a very low place" [CAN].

Such genuine caring provides an aspirational model for public healthcare service in Hong Kong. Here, we will quote one interview passage that did not share any themes with other interviews and hence has not yet appeared in this book to demonstrate this point further, because this passage shows a scenario opposite to genuine caring. After one interviewee at first said that she could not think of a significant enough response for the final set interview question (which asks interviewees to recount a particularly impactful experience in their career), she reached out again to the interviewer to share her views the next day. She described an encounter between a patient and a senior doctor that she witnessed in her "first year in this specialty":

> The patient's condition was a little bit poor. […] She had come in for a surgery. […] I'm guessing that [the senior doctor] thought that she had to give a bit of a warning to the patient because her condition was bad. […] So she told the patient—and this is something I remember to this day […]: "Old lady, you will die. You're in great danger, do you realize this? You will die." The lady burst into tears. Yes, I remember this incident really well. […]
>
> Now after working for so many years, I think back and I realize that [the patient's] condition was only a bit bad, not very bad. But maybe that "senior" [doctor] thought that it would be

> safest to describe [the surgery] as dangerously as possible. [...] The patient was okay in the end. But she was very scared. [CAN]

The safety that senior doctor prioritized was not that of the patient, but her own. The interviewee vowed "never to become a person like that" who would "talk like that to a patient" [CAN]. This example provides a stark contrast to the interview narratives we have read so far that describe how challenging it can be—especially in the time allowed for patients in the Hong Kong public hospital setting—for doctors to work towards an ethics of care that is not coldly clinical but warmly clinical, allowing empathy, humanity, and emotions their place while retaining the professionalism that is necessary in a healthcare setting. Different doctors thought differently about the extent of empathy and emotional engagement needed, and how they could allow these to shape the clinical encounter. However, interviewees' descriptions of these struggles and of how they developed their own solutions to them show the importance of these ingredients to care instead of mere "care behavior" and what Marcum (2012) termed "uncaring" (p. 132), so vividly exemplified in the passage just quoted. They remind us not to neglect these components in public hospital care in Hong Kong—even while continuing the important push for efficiency based on analyses and projections of population composition and resources to address the problems in the sector.

3.5 Closing Remarks

Doctors' narratives of work were collated in this book to document and gain an understanding of doctors' lived experience of their work in public hospitals in Hong Kong, and as portraits of their working lives. The resultant alternative understanding of doctors' public hospital work may or may not form the basis for future changes from a health policy perspective—and indeed, to aim directly for these was not this study's primary goal, as the Introduction explained—but it is hoped that hearing doctors narrate the realities of their work can resonate deeply with a wide variety of readers. For doctors and doctors-in-training, the resonance of shared experience can offer some companionship and guidance, perhaps to—even if only momentarily—pause automatic engagement with work. This can open up the space for deeper reflection on whether and how the shared experiences apply to them, and for possible ways to personally modify the meanings and values that interviewees described. This may also provide them with a broader range of starting points from which to explore, for themselves, how to nurture an improved and healthier fit between the self and work, for a more sustaining career in the public hospital sector in Hong Kong. For the public, reading about the experiences of and problems faced by some of the doctors whom they may encounter in public hospitals when they or their loved ones fall ill could lead to better mutual understanding, perhaps attenuating some of the antipathy that can result due to what the public regards as inadequate medical services, poor "staff attitudes," and frustrating wait times (Cheung, 2023; Siu, 2019). And when news stories in Hong Kong on serious problems in the public health sector appear—as they do on a regular basis, with the *South China Morning Post*'s year-end review of all the high-profile medical blunders in December 2024 (Heung, 2024) serving as a prominent recent example—taking doctors' narratives into consideration may encourage additional ways of reacting to and thinking about these issues. In this way, resonating with the meanings, ideals, motivations, emotions, and anxieties—or to summarize in one word, humanity—behind the work of the public hospital doctor in Hong Kong encourages new and different ways of looking at their work that could, in future, allow it to be shaped more humanely, for both the doctor and the patient.

References

Avrahami, E. (2011). Positive wrongdoings: Reading doctors' narratives on ordinary ethics. *Literature and Medicine, 29*(2), 325–354. https://doi.org/10.1353/lm.2011.0327

Bennett, D., Solomon, Y., Bergin, C., Horgan, M., & Dornan, T. (2017). Possibility and agency in Figured Worlds: Becoming a "good doctor." *Medical Education, 51*(3), 248–257. https://doi.org/10.1111/medu.13220

Busireddy, K. R., Miller, J. A., Ellison, K., Ren, V., Qayyum, R., & Panda, M. (2017). Efficacy of interventions to reduce resident physician burnout: A systematic review. *Journal of Graduate Medical Education, 9*(3), 294–301. https://doi.org/10.4300/JGME-D-16-00372.1

Chang, Y. K., Oh, W.-Y., & Han, S. (2022). Profit or purpose: What increases medical doctors' job satisfaction? *Healthcare, 10*(4), 641. https://doi.org/10.3390/healthcare10040641

Charon, R. (2011). The novelization of the body, or, how medicine and stories need one another. *Narrative, 19*(1), 33–50. https://doi.org/10.1353/nar.2011.0004

Cheung, E. (2023, December 11). Hong Kong public hospital complaints go up 33%; user appreciation falls 12.4%. *South China Morning Post*. https://www.scmp.com/news/hong-kong/health-environment/article/3244715/hong-kong-public-hospitals-see-complaints-rise-third-public-appreciation-drops-124

Fisher, J., Cuff, P., Couper, I., von Pressentin, K., Strasser, R., Green-Thompson, L., & Aparna, R. (2022). The social determinants of lifelong learning. In S. C. Scrimshaw, Sandra D. Lane, R. A. Rubinstein, & J. Fisher (Eds.), *The SAGE handbook of social studies in health and medicine* (2nd ed., pp. 631–649). Sage.

Green-Thompson, L. P., McInerney, P., & Woollard, B. (2017). The social accountability of doctors: A relationship based framework for understanding emergent community concepts of caring. *BMC Health Services Research, 17*, 269. https://doi.org/10.1186/s12913-017-2239-7

Halpern, J. (2003). What is clinical empathy? *Journal of General Internal Medicine, 18*(8), 670–674. https://doi.org/10.1046/j.1525-1497.2003.21017.x

Health Bureau. (2023, February 1). *Develop a community-based primary healthcare system*. https://www.primaryhealthcare.gov.hk/bp/en/supplementary-documents/develop-a-community-based-system/

Heung, S. (2024, December 28). Hong Kong's year in medical blunders, from unneeded surgery to detached tubes. *South China Morning Post*. https://www.scmp.com/news/hong-kong/health-environment/article/3292585/hong-kongs-year-medical-blunders-unneeded-surgery-detached-tubes

Irvine, C., & Charon, R. (2017). Deliver us from certainty: Training for narrative ethics. In R. Charon, S. DasGupta, N. Hermann, C. Irvine, E. Marcus, E. Rivera Colón, D. Spencer, & M. Spiegel (Eds.), *The principles and practice of narrative medicine* (pp. 110–133). Oxford University Press.

Irvine, C., & Spencer, D. (2017). Dualism and its discontents: Philosophy, literature, and medicine. In R. Charon, S. DasGupta, N. Hermann, C. Irvine, E. Marcus, E. Rivera Colón, D. Spencer, & M. Spiegel (Eds.), *The principles and practice of narrative medicine* (pp. 63–86). Oxford University Press.

Lam, D. T. Y. (2024). Three critical elements of sustainable healthcare. In *Building a sustainable healthcare system for Hong Kong* (pp. 11–26). The Hong Kong institute of Asia-Pacific Studies, The Chinese University of Hong Kong. https://www.hkiaps.cuhk.edu.hk/wp-content/uploads/2024/07/PRR07.pdf

Marcum, J. A. (2012). *The virtuous physician: The role of virtue in medicine*. Springer.

Mason, A. (2000). *Community, solidarity and belonging: Levels of community and their normative significance*. Cambridge University Press.

Moore, J. (2009). A consideration of the qualities of a "good" doctor with some help from the humanities. *The British Journal of General Practice: THe Journal of the Royal College of General Practitioners, 59*(558), 58–61. https://doi.org/10.3399/bjgp09X394950

See, K. C., Zhao, M. Y., Nakataki, E., Chittawatanarat, K., Fang, W. F., Faruq, M. O., Wahjuprajitno, B., Arabi, Y. M., Wong, W. T., Divatia, J. V., Palo, J. E., Shrestha, B. R., Nafees, K. M. K., Binh, N. G., Al Rahma, H. N., Detleuxay, K., Ong, V., Phua, J., & SABA Study Investigators and the Asian Critical Care Clinical Trials Group. (2018). Professional burnout among physicians and nurses in Asian intensive care units: A multinational survey. *Intensive Care Medicine, 44*(12), 2079–2090. https://doi.org/10.1007/s00134-018-5432-1

Siu, C. F. Y., Yuen, S. K., & Cheung, A. (2012). Burnout among public doctors in Hong Kong: Cross-sectional survey. *Hong Kong Medical Journal, 18*, 186–92. https://www.hkmj.org/system/files/hkm1206p186.pdf

Siu, P. (2019, May 19). Just one-third of Hong Kong residents satisfied with public hospital services as long waiting times and lack of care top list of gripes. *South China Morning Post*. https://www.scmp.com/news/hong-kong/health-environment/article/3010839/just-one-third-hong-kong-residents-satisfied

Spiegel, M., & Spencer, D. (2017a). Accounts of self: Exploring relationality through literature. In R. Charon, S. DasGupta, N. Hermann, C. Irvine, E. Marcus, E. Rivera Colón, D. Spencer, & M. Spiegel (Eds.), *The principles and practice of narrative medicine* (pp. 15–36). Oxford University Press.

Spiegel, M., & Spencer, D. (2017b). This is what we do, and these things happen: Literature, experience, emotion, and relationality in the classroom. In R. Charon, S. DasGupta, N. Hermann, C. Irvine, E. Marcus, E. Rivera Colón, D. Spencer, & M. Spiegel (Eds.), *The principles and practice of narrative medicine* (pp. 37–59). Oxford University Press.

West, C. P., Dyrbye, L. N., & Shanafelt, T. D. (2018). Physician burnout: Contributors, consequences and solutions. *Journal of Internal Medicine, 283*(6), 516–529. https://doi.org/10.1111/joim.12752

Yuen, P. P. (2024). Financing sustainable healthcare systems. In *Building a sustainable healthcare system for Hong Kong* (pp. 102–118). The Hong Kong institute of Asia-Pacific Studies, The Chinese University of Hong Kong. https://www.hkiaps.cuhk.edu.hk/wp-content/uploads/2024/07/PRR07.pdf

The manufacturer's authorised representative in the EU is Springer Nature Customer Service Centre GmbH, Europaplatz 3, 69115 Heidelberg, Germany. If you have any concerns regarding our products, please contact ProductSafety@springernature.com

Printed and bound by CPI Group (UK) Ltd, Croydon, CR0 4YY
01/10/2026
02225944-0005